# SHATTERED

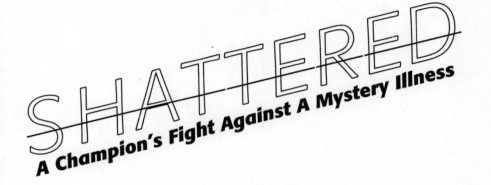

# SHATTERED

## A Champion's Fight Against A Mystery Illness

# PETER MARSHALL
## WITH NICK KEHOE

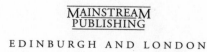

MAINSTREAM
PUBLISHING

EDINBURGH AND LONDON

First published in Great Britain in 2001 by
MAINSTREAM PUBLISHING COMPANY (EDINBURGH) LTD
7 Albany Street
Edinburgh EH1 3UG

ISBN 1 84018 395 0

A catalogue record for this book is available
from the British Library

Typeset in 10 on 12pt Apollo
Printed and bound in Great Britain by
Butler and Tanner Ltd, Frome and London

# CONTENTS

| | | |
|---|---|---|
| | FOREWORD BY JONAH BARRINGTON | 7 |
| | INTRODUCTION | 11 |
| 1 | HUMILIATED | 15 |
| 2 | MIGHTY MOUSE | 27 |
| 3 | THE NEW KID ON THE BLOCK | 43 |
| 4 | BEATING KING KHAN | 59 |
| 5 | THE EASTERN MASTER | 77 |
| 6 | ILL? BUT YOU DON'T LOOK ILL! | 95 |
| 7 | FOR LOVE OR MONEY | 109 |
| 8 | A LIFE MORE ORDINARY | 121 |
| 9 | WINNING THE WORLD CUP | 133 |
| 10 | THE BIGGER PICTURE | 145 |
| 11 | MIND GAMES | 159 |
| 12 | A KINDER WAY TO FITNESS | 175 |
| 13 | BRITISH CHAMPION AGAIN | 187 |
| | POSTSCRIPT | 201 |
| | DAILY SUMMER TRAINING AND COMPETITION PLANNER | 205 |

# FOREWORD

When I think of Peter Marshall's story I find it hard not to get angry. The man is truly amazing, but he has been treated very shabbily. To battle through four years of debilitating illness and then come back to demolish some of the best players in the world is a wonderful achievement. It would have been astonishing if someone had done it in darts or snooker; to do it in a high-energy sport like squash is scarcely believable. Disappointingly, Peter has had to battle not only with his illness but also with the stupidity and prejudice of people who should have been there to support him. There are many doctors and journalists who should feel ashamed. In the end, perhaps their lack of understanding doesn't matter, for Peter succeeded without them. In doing so, he's provided us with the most remarkable and inspiring sports story of the last ten years. Anyone who knows this formidable character as well as I do will be delighted he came through. No one, however, will be in the least surprised, for he has an iron will.

I first met Peter when he was only eight years old. His squash coach had asked me if I would take a look at this curious little fellow who'd been mowing down players twice his age. Peter was so tiny I nicknamed him Mighty Mouse. He wasn't strong enough to hold the heavy wooden racket properly, so he played two-handed. I went on court expecting a gentle knock around and was amazed at what I saw. He hit the ball like an arrow down both wings, very fast and with incredible accuracy, and had a stronger basic game and a greater understanding of squash than any kid I'd ever seen. I went home thinking that I had met someone very special.

My initial impression was reinforced every time I met Peter over the following years as he advanced through the junior ranks. I coached him at numerous national squad sessions, and was always impressed by his talent and dedication. He matured into a world-class performer, and by the age of

7

23 the world of squash was his for the taking. Then came the onset of chronic fatigue syndrome. It's a measure of his willpower that despite feeling tired and lethargic he played on for a year before his health finally gave way. Had he remained fit, there is no doubt in my mind that Peter would have become world number one and dominated the game for several years.

Sadly, those precious years were spent in a fruitless search for a cure. His plight wasn't helped by the prejudice surrounding chronic fatigue syndrome, with many people in the medical profession and the media dismissing it as some sort of yuppie ailment that was all in the mind. It made me angry to read so much garbage written by people who should have known better, yet seemed to make a living from knocking the sick. Peter had to endure endless sessions with doctors and experts who, at best, were powerless to help him; at worst, they were unsympathetic and too quick to dismiss his condition as purely psychological. I remember recoiling in horror when I heard he'd been prescribed some very potent anti-depressants. I got on the phone to him straight away and told him to stop taking them.

There is no way that Peter's illness could be dismissed as some sort of mental weakness: there is nothing in his background to substantiate such a claim. Psychologically, he was as hard as nails – so much so that he reached the final of the British Open at a time when he was seriously ill. I remember him telling me that he was experiencing excruciating pain in the area of his liver. He felt as though he'd been kicked by a horse. In spite of this, he soldiered on and produced some wonderful squash. I have never known anyone who could suppress pain and discomfort as well as he could. Ironically, it was probably this capacity to take physical punishment that drove him further into the illness.

It is wrong that a sportsman of the calibre of Peter Marshall should be treated in this way: we don't have many world-class sportsmen in this country, so when we find the genuine article we ought to treat them better. As it was, Peter drifted into a sporting wilderness in which he was left to fend for himself. It was pot luck whether or not he would happen to walk through the door of a doctor who was both sympathetic to his plight and able to help him. It's hard to imagine stars of equal calibre in other sports such as football, people like David Beckham or Michael Owen, being left to their own devices in this way.

It was perhaps the lack of proper guidance that led Peter to make a comeback attempt in 1997 after two years out of the game. Such was his talent that despite having done little training, he was still able to outplay the hottest property on the circuit at that time, Jonathan Power. Unfortunately, his illness was still there and he had to withdraw. His second comeback in 1999 was far more successful. Although he might still have had the illness within his system, Peter had learnt a lot and was better able to manage his health and career – he set about overpowering some of the best players around, won his first two tournaments, became British National Champion and zoomed into the top ten. It was wonderful to see.

———————

One can scarcely imagine the mental trauma Peter went through as his illness took hold. How did he cope with not knowing what was wrong with him? With the fear that he might never know, and might never be well? How did he face the prejudice invoked by chronic fatigue syndrome? And what about the frustration of watching lesser players usurp his position at the top? I don't know how he did it, but I do know he had to reach for strength deep within himself. There was little help from outside.

Peter once told me that as a boy he saw all the British Open titles I had won and was inspired to do the same himself. Well, now it seems the tables have turned; I'm the one gaining inspiration from him. I recently had a hip replacement operation, and sometimes wonder if I should still be playing squash. Then I look at what Peter has overcome and I think: 'Of course I should. If he can play after all he's been through, then I can too.' I think many other people will gain inspiration in the same way. Not just those trying to overcome chronic fatigue syndrome, but anyone who has allowed obstacles to prevent them achieving their own secret Everest.

Wherever we are, and no matter how old we are, we all need something to stimulate us and drive us on that bit further. I can think of very few things more likely to do that than the story of Peter Marshall.

*Jonah Barrington*
*November 2000*

# INTRODUCTION

It was an embarrassing moment for me, but the police were very understanding under the circumstances. I had gone away for the weekend and, in an absentminded way that my friends tell me is typical, I left my front door wide open. After a day or so my neighbours became worried and knocked on the door to see if I was all right. When there was no answer, they stepped inside to see if there was any sign of life. They were horrified to find that the place had apparently been ransacked – there were clothes and papers and goodness knows what scattered all over the floor. The neighbours phoned the police immediately to report that my house had been burgled and left in a dreadful state. I was finally tracked down and returned home straight away, hoping that nothing valuable had been taken.

I needn't have worried. When I got back, I found that everything was just as I had left it. I felt very sheepish, and had to admit to the police that my house always looked like this. It might have appeared chaotic to other people, but to me it was in perfect order. Yes, I'm afraid it was just like the TV advert for *Yellow Pages*. The police saw the funny side of it eventually, but I felt very guilty for having wasted their time.

Apart from the embarrassment, the episode was of no particular significance to me. My friends think otherwise. To them, it's a perfect example of what they see as the chaos which pervades my personal life, as opposed to the total discipline and focus which characterises my approach to my job as a professional squash player. The Scottish player Martin Heath regards me as something of an English eccentric and delights in what he considers to be my idiosyncrasies. He says he's constantly amazed at how I can be walking along absentmindedly at a big tournament with my shoelaces undone, spilling coffee on my shirt and talking about any

11

old thing. Then, moments later, when I walk onto the court to play, everything changes. Suddenly I become totally organised, totally focused. My concentration is absolute. Martin thinks this is because it is only when I get on court that everything finally makes sense to me and I become the master of my own fate.

This may be overstating the case a little and I'm probably more organised than people might think, but Martin has a point. In my early days, my life did revolve around building my career and it took up most of my thinking. You have to work hard to get to the top in any profession and it's fair to say that I probably worked harder than most. I put myself through years of punishing training routines and for a while everything seemed to be going fine. By the time I was 23, I had got to number two in the world and immediately set my sights on taking the top spot. That was no small task. It meant overtaking the man I regard as the best player the world has ever seen, Jansher Khan. At that time, in the early to mid-'90s, he was way ahead of all challengers and in no mood for being overtaken by anybody.

Nevertheless, I believed I would eventually replace him and set about making it happen as quickly as possible. I trained harder than ever and spent hours on court honing my skills. I was happy to stay on long after everyone else had gone. It worked, for a while at least, and I became one of the fittest sportsmen in the world. I was also very strong mentally. I would never give in until the last drop of energy was gone. I became renowned for my indomitable spirit, so much so that I think some players were intimidated before they even stepped on court with me. They knew they would have to give everything they had and more to beat me. Some players weren't always ready to do that.

The England star Simon Parke has been one of my best friends since childhood, and knows me better than anyone else in the game. When he's in a polite mood he describes me as one of the mentally strongest people he's ever met. When he's in a less refined mood, he uses phrases like 'absolute animal' and 'stubborn bastard' to describe me. Whatever words he uses, it amounts to the same thing. I was ferocious in my determination to succeed. Perhaps too ferocious for my own good, as it turned out.

Jansher Khan remained frustratingly hard to catch no matter what I did. Many players would have accepted that he was in a class of his own and congratulated themselves on doing so well in getting to the world number two slot, then settled down to enjoy their careers and the very seductive lifestyle that goes along with being a professional sportsman. Not me, though. That wasn't my way at all. I could never settle for second best and wanted to become the world number one. Even more than that, perhaps, I wanted to rise to the challenge of beating Jansher. If Jansher had retired and allowed me to assume the top slot, I wouldn't have been satisfied – I would have felt a little flat. I had to beat him if being world champion was really to mean something. This wasn't because I had anything personal against Jansher; it's just that he was the best and I wanted to prove myself against him. There was an indefinable yet irresistible attraction in reaching a level where I could play the best squash in the world and surpass the best player in the world. Maybe there was something too pure, too perfectionist in that desire.

Whatever the case, my response to suffering several drubbings at the hands of the master was to train harder and concentrate even more on the task in hand. I had a certain amount of success. I closed the gap between us enormously and became the only player in the world who could test him. I gave him several frights and took him to numerous nailbiting five-set matches in major finals all over the world. I eventually reached a stage where I felt sure that within our next few meetings I would beat him and start to gain the ascendancy. I was approaching my peak, and he would surely have to start going downhill soon.

He did start to fade a few years later, but by then it was too late for me. I had crashed out of the game suffering from something I had hardly even heard of at that time, chronic fatigue syndrome. It blew my life apart and left me battered and bewildered. Instead of being the fittest player on the circuit, able to slug it out with anyone for hours on end, I was finding it difficult to walk upstairs. The physical pain was nothing compared with the mental anguish. I lost the best years of my career. I had to lie back while players I used to beat quite easily went on to take over from Jansher and dominate the game. Doctors couldn't point to any definite cure. I would rest for months, yet feel no better. My emotions were all over the place as I wrestled with the problem of how to regain some control over my life.

It led me to a four-year odyssey where I had to look closely at myself and work out what had gone wrong. What was this chronic fatigue syndrome? Was it a physical thing? Was it psychological? Was it a mixture of both? It was easy to pose the questions but much harder to find the answers. In the end, I had to work most of it out for myself. I happen to be a squash player and so my experiences come mainly from my sport. However, I think a lot of what led me to become ill is common to sufferers in many other walks of life. That doesn't mean everything I did will apply to them, but I think many people will recognise in their own experiences the feelings I had and the mistakes I made as I tried to get to the top.

In those early days, my strength also turned out to be my weakness. I did too much and my body eventually rebelled. Paradoxically, the same strength that got me into trouble may also have got me out again. Even when my illness was at its worst, I refused to give in and eventually worked my way back. I'm not saying that what worked for me will work for everyone, but hopefully it will show people what can be achieved. As for me, I just want to enjoy the rest of my career and hopefully pick up a few of the trophies I missed out on first time round. I'm a lot more relaxed about it now, however. All well and good if it happens for me, but if it doesn't I won't worry too much. I still want to do well but I now have a broader perspective.

My illness has been painful and it still hurts to think I'll never be able to get back what should have been the best years of my career. There are compensations, however. I've become a very different animal to the one Simon described in the early part of my career. I now feel I'm a more rounded person with a more realistic grip on what is and isn't important in life. I'm not saying I've totally beaten chronic fatigue syndrome, but I have managed to rebuild my career and I'm reasonably confident for the future. It's great to be back working again, a huge boost to my self-esteem after spending so long feeling I had been thrown on the scrap heap. I might never be as good as I could have been, but I must be doing something right because I've forced my way back among the world's top ten and won several tournaments. More importantly, my health is holding up and I'm enjoying life.

Not only that, but my house is a lot tidier now and I usually remember to lock the door when I go out.

# 1.
## HUMILIATED

My dad was the first person to notice that something was wrong. The problem had been creeping up on me for nearly a year. Sometimes I might be a little sluggish on court and would dismiss it as an off-day. Or I might feel a little more tired than usual after a tournament and would tell myself that I wasn't fit enough – I needed to train harder. Then the off-days became more frequent. The tiredness became more severe, and it became harder to explain it away. Something was happening, but I didn't know what. I tried to put it out of my mind. Then, in April 1995, I played Mark Cairns in the second round of the British Open. I won relatively easily but I didn't feel well. Dad came to see me after the game and asked me if I was all right. He said I didn't look my normal self on court. I wasn't so full of life.

That was when I first told him I had been suffering a strange form of tiredness that sometimes overwhelmed me. I'd been to see several doctors, but none of them seemed to know what was wrong. The previous June my GP suggested that I had been overdoing things a bit and needed to take more rest. He recommended that I cut down on training for a month and see how I felt then. I did as he said, but taking things easy was a hard concept for me to grasp. I was rising up the world rankings and didn't want anything to stop my progress. I was only 23. I wanted to push on.

By August, I felt a bit better and so I increased my training to prepare for the new season. Things went well and within the next few months I got to number two in the world. Only the legendary Jansher Khan was ahead of me. I should have been elated, but I wasn't. The lethargy kept coming back and it was getting worse every time. It was particularly bad in January and February and, on the doctor's advice, I had stopped training again for nearly a month. I couldn't rest much longer because I had to prepare for the British Open.

After keeping it to myself for so long it was a relief to tell someone. My dad looked worried. He had always put my wellbeing first and my squash career second. But what could he say? It was hard for him to give advice when we didn't yet know what we were up against. Eventually, he said that if I felt really bad then I should pull out of the tournament. But if possible, it might be better to struggle on and then sort out the fatigue problem afterwards. That is what I decided to do. I got through the next round and then met Brett Martin in the semi-final. I had played him several times over the years and the games were always hard because he was such a skillful and deceptive player. I won, but he fought me all the way and it took a lot out of me physically. I wasn't too worried: I expected to recover by the following day, and I had the prospect of yet another final against Jansher Khan to inspire me.

Within an hour of coming off court, however, I knew that something was wrong. I felt drained. As I walked upstairs after dinner my legs felt heavy as lead. I sat in my hotel room feeling uneasy and apprehensive. I was worse than I had ever been before, but I didn't know why. It didn't make sense. I was a fiercely fit athlete in one of the most demanding sports of all, and was known as one of the strongest players on the circuit. I was used to pushing my body to its limits in gruelling training sessions and marathon matches that could last for over two hours. My stamina was one of my main weapons. Now just walking across the room seemed an effort.

Even more worrying was what was going on in my mind. Normally I would be excited and full of enthusiasm on the eve of an important match. Yet here I was about to play one of the biggest games of my life and I felt totally listless. There was no sense of occasion at all. Tomorrow could have been just another day, rather than the day on which I was to take on the greatest player in the world, possibly the greatest player ever. In those days, very few things could excite an up-and-coming squash player more than the prospect of battling with Jansher Khan. From the moment he inherited the crown of his countryman and namesake, Jahingir Khan, he straddled the sport like a colossus, taking on the world's best players and beating them all. Such was his dominance that he hardly ever lost. In the early '90s, I think I can honestly say I was getting closer to him than anyone else in the world. He was quoted at the time as saying this about me: 'Peter is very fit and never gives up. I know he is the biggest danger to me.' I played him numerous times over a four-year period and had beaten him twice in club matches, but never in a major final. That was what I really wanted.

As I sat in that hotel room in Cardiff, I knew the scene was set for me to go that extra mile the next day and claim a victory on a world stage. The British Open was the most prestigious tournament of them all, squash's equivalent to Wimbledon. I had first gone there as a star-struck fan at the age of 11 with my parents. We'd been every year since. I had seen all the greats, like Jahingir Khan, Rodney Martin, Chris Dittmar and of course Jansher Khan. When I became a player at the age of 17, the British Open retained its special status for me. I always looked forward to it more than any other tournament. Now I had progressed from teenage fan and apprentice player to a genuine contender for the title. I had everything to play for. I was the first British player to reach the final of the British Open since Jonah Barrington. And if you class Jonah as Irish, as he really was even though he spent most of his life in England, then I was the first Englishman ever to reach the final.

Many people thought I could do it. Some expected it. I got loads of good luck messages, more than I had received for any match before. Everyone in England and most neutrals from other countries wanted me to win. Not because they had anything against Jansher; it was more to do with the fact that, through him and Jahingir, the name Khan had appeared on the trophy for around 15 years and it was time for a change. I desperately wanted to be the one to change it. I knew I could do it. The gap between us was narrowing. A few months earlier I had pushed Jansher all the way in front of his home crowd in the final of the Pakistan Open.

Squash is very popular in Pakistan, where the top players are household names and are treated like superstars. Jansher had an army of fans who were fanatical in their support. They were much more vociferous during games than the more reserved observers I was used to back home in England. They yelled and willed Jansher on during my epic final with him. They didn't have any effect on me, though, and I played some of the best squash of my life. It was a titanic battle and I loved every second of it. I eventually lost, but it was 3–2 and frighteningly close. I think Jansher knew it could have gone either way. This time, in front of my home crowd,

I felt I could go one better. My family and friends thought so too and many of them had travelled down from Nottingham to Cardiff to support me. They might not shout as loud as Jansher's followers in Pakistan, but their presence would still be a help. The situation couldn't have been better except for one thing. I felt terrible.

I told myself not to worry as I went to bed that night. I reassured myself that I would feel much better in the morning and lay down fully expecting to have a restless night; it's usually hard to sleep well before a big final. There's too much tension and excitement in the air. That night, though, I felt little excitement and slept surprisingly well. I didn't wake up until eight the next morning and after such a good night's sleep, I should have felt great. I didn't. I was still tired and lethargic. It was worrying, but I tried not to admit it to myself. I wanted to remain positive.

I went straight down to the practice court to do a little light work and tried to block all negative thoughts from my mind. While going through some set routines on my own, I felt I was hitting the ball quite well but didn't seem to have any spark. I was worried. I only stayed for about 20 minutes and then went to get some breakfast. Afterwards I went back to my hotel room and tried to make sense of what was happening. The whole tournament had been a huge struggle for me. There was too much dependence on adrenaline and determination. The semi-final against Brett Martin had been hard, but not that hard. I had played many tough games over the years and normally recovered very quickly. I would certainly be back to normal by the following day. Not this time. My legs and my whole body felt very heavy, and I was having pains under my liver; there was a stabbing sensation in my left-hand side. It just wasn't normal. Surely this was more serious than the doctors had thought. Perhaps they had missed something?

As the morning wore on, it became clear that I wasn't likely to get any better before the match that evening. I would have to go on court feeling like this. I didn't know if I could get through it. The prospect of playing Jansher didn't worry me, and never had – there was never any pressure because he was always the favourite; just being able to give him a good game was considered an achievement. I would normally relish the opportunity to test myself against him, but this time I was worried about not being able to do myself justice. People had come a long way and hopes were high. What if I let everyone down?

Normally, I wouldn't have to psyche myself up for such an important game but I did on this occasion. I told myself to put all my worries out of my mind. Treat it as just another game. I just needed to hold myself together for another few hours. It didn't matter that I felt terrible. If I could just push myself on now, then I could rest afterwards. Everything would be fine. I settled down to relax by listening to some music. I liked the Chemical Brothers and put one of their tapes in my Walkman, but still felt restless so I started browsing through magazines and flicking through the TV channels. Nothing could take my mind off the way I was feeling. Instead, I decided to focus on the match.

I always like to set aside at least half an hour to work out my game plan for whoever I'm playing. All squash players have their own particular style which they stick to as much as possible, but it's always a good idea to analyse the other person's strengths and weaknesses and adjust if you think it might give you an advantage. The problem with Jansher was that he was nearly all strengths and virtually no weaknesses. He tended to dominate the T very well, and as all club squash players know, that is where so many games are won and lost. He was also a few years older and more experienced, so he was better at changing tactics than I was. He was the ultimate squash player.

I still felt I could beat him, however. He was declining physically and mentally, and he could get upset if things weren't going his way. He had been known to get downhearted and his concentration could waver. Jansher liked a slow game, allowing himself plenty of time to play his shots. I thought my best tactic therefore was to keep the pace up as much as possible. When I had beaten him in the club matches I had played a very fast game, taking the ball early and stopping him from settling into his normal routine.

As I sat there wondering about the British Open final, I decided I would take the same approach. I felt that if I could force him to play long rallies then his mind might wander a little and I could move in for the kill. The other advantage of keeping the rallies long was that it would play to my strength, my great fitness. Jansher had tremendous stamina, but I thought I had even more. Or I had until now. That day, I wasn't very confident my stamina would hold up at all. Nevertheless, that had to be my game plan. It was the only way I would have any chance.

With the tactics decided, I tried to put the match completely out of my mind and went to have lunch with my dad. He knew I was still feeling unwell but neither of us wanted to talk about it at that stage. It was important to focus on the game. I told him about the way I intended to play and he was very encouraging. I got back to the hotel room at about three o'clock. I just wanted to rest. I lay down for an hour but had to start getting ready for the game at four. It was important to start psyching myself up, because I wasn't feeling very enthusiastic. I had to keep reminding myself that this was the final of the biggest squash tournament in the world. I started checking through my gear, just for something to do – I made sure I had all five rackets, three or four spare shirts and so on.

At about six o'clock I went down to the courts. They were only a two-minute walk from the hotel. The women's final was being played, so I stopped to watch for a while just to get the atmosphere of the place. Naturally, people started to talk to me so I went to the dressing rooms at the back of the courts. It's not that I'm unsociable. It's just that you don't want any distractions in the run-up to a big game; you want to focus purely on the task ahead. Unfortunately, I wasn't feeling any better. I tried to block it from my mind. There was no time to worry about my health. Before a big game you don't want to admit to any weaknesses, not even to yourself. I had to be positive no matter what. I reminded myself of the Pakistan Open six months earlier when I had run Jansher so close and nearly stolen it from him. That buoyed me up for a moment or two, but I couldn't deceive myself for long. During the Pakistan Open, I had been fit and fresh and hungry to play. I felt I could run forever. This time, I felt I could hardly run at all.

About half an hour before the match, I went out to warm up. You can usually tell from the warm-up how you're feeling. I was hitting the ball reasonably well, but mentally I was finding it difficult to get started. It was an effort to go through the usual simple routines. It occurred to me that I ought to be feeling more excited about this game than anything I had done before. Somehow I wasn't – it all seemed a bit flat. The same negative thoughts kept entering my mind. I tried to push myself, because it was getting nearer to the start of the match and the adrenaline was starting to flow. I perked up a little. I kept telling myself to put everything aside and really go for it. Rest could come afterwards.

At about ten to seven, the compère came into the dressing room and asked me and Jansher to stand at the entrance to the court. He introduced us to the audience and listed all our major achievements. There were thousands of people watching. I could see my family and some of my friends from Nottingham. That gave me a lift. Then they switched off the lights and put on the music as we walked onto the court. It was the kind of big occasion I loved and gave me a tremendous boost. Jansher and I took off our tracksuits and started knocking up. Suddenly, the hunger and enthusiasm I had been seeking all day came flooding back. As we went through the warm-up rallies, I was getting really psyched up. I couldn't wait to start the game. Maybe I was going to be all right after all. I felt a sense of relief and a surge of confidence. Perhaps the big occasion was going to save me. Perhaps I would be able to perform after all.

Within three rallies, that newfound hope was shattered. I had never felt so bad on a squash court. I had never felt so bad anywhere. I wasn't breathing very well, but the most noticeable thing was how much my muscles were aching. It was as if I was producing lots of lactic acid very early on and my limbs felt heavy. My whole body was lethargic. There was no energy. My coordination and movement were totally out. Deep down, I knew there was no way I could win. I was struggling. I couldn't turn it round. My carefully thought out game plan was coming to nothing. I kept urging myself on, but every movement required a huge act of will. I kept going through pure determination and a dread of letting people down. I lost the first three points and took a real hammering throughout the first game. It ended 15–4, and I still don't know how I managed to get four.

My England team-mate Simon Parke, an old friend since schooldays and in the world top ten, had come along to advise me between games. If anyone could gee me up it would be him. He told me to forget about the first game and to play as if we were starting from scratch. He urged me on and pointed out that the match was far from over. There was still plenty of time for a comeback. I told him I had no energy at all. There was little he or anyone could say to remedy that. Simon tried to advise me on tactical changes to hurt Jansher more, but I wasn't able to take much of it in. I was too concerned about how I was going to find the strength to carry on.

We went back on court and in the first rally I made a big effort to get back into it and maybe turn things round. It was no good. I was still miles off the pace. Jansher was playing as well as I expected. He was volleying superbly and taking everything early. I felt helpless. Normally, if you get off to a bad start or you're not playing well you try to change things around a bit; alter your tactics by making the rallies last longer or perhaps going for a winner much earlier. But I couldn't do anything. It was an unnerving experience. On a squash court you're surrounded by four glass walls. I felt I was trapped, with no escape. Beyond the walls, I was aware of thousands of pairs of eyes looking down on me scrutinising my every move. I could sense people wondering what on earth was going on. Why was I playing in such a feeble way? It was embarrassing and I felt so alone. There was nowhere to hide. It wasn't like a team game where I could seek anonymity in numbers.

There was nothing I could do but soldier on. It was hopeless. I just couldn't perform at all. I lost 15–4 again. It was the same story in the third game. I was feeling even more tired and went down 15–5. I was devastated. It was my worst ever performance. I had never been beaten so easily before. The match only lasted about 35 minutes. I had been run ragged and made to look like a novice rather than the second-best player in the world. I had never before felt so disappointed and angry after losing. I remained painfully aware of those thousands of eyes still glaring down at me, puzzling over my total inability to fulfil their expectations. Jansher shook my hand but he didn't say anything. I don't know if he suspected something was wrong but he must have been surprised by my lack of resistance, especially as we had been so close in previous matches.

As soon as the game was over, Jansher fell to his knees and kissed the floor as he always did after a major victory. His entourage of fans rushed onto the court to join him. They were shouting and celebrating a great victory for their hero. Unfortunately, the smaller yet equally loyal band of family and friends who had come to support me had far less to cheer about. I felt I had let them down and was furious with myself. How could I have let it happen? I felt humiliated. Disgraced. I had played in front of a huge home crowd who all believed in me and I hadn't been able to reach anything like my true potential. I walked straight off court and couldn't speak to anyone. The TV and newspaper reporters wanted to do interviews and normally I'm fine with things like that, whether I've won or lost. But not this time – I just couldn't face it. I brushed past the press and cameramen and went straight to my hotel room.

I sat there and started to berate myself. I had just been in the final of the British Open Championship, my ambition since childhood. What could be better than to play in the game's greatest tournament against the game's greatest player? Yet when the opportunity came, I hadn't been able to perform. The frustration was driving me mad. However, under the anger there was another emotion – fear. Although I was being hard on myself, I knew that it wasn't really my fault. This was getting serious. Something was wrong. Something I didn't understand.

Dad and a few close friends came to the room and tried to cheer me up. They knew I hadn't been 100 per cent and told me not to worry. There would be another chance soon. I nodded my agreement and, at the time, I thought they were right. Over the last few years I had got used to meeting Jansher in the finals of the game's biggest tournaments. It wasn't something I took for granted, but we had pulled away from the rest of the pack. I was the only one really pushing him. I fully expected that once this disappointment was behind me, I would be back playing him again within a few months, in another big match. Maybe then I would win and regain some of my self-respect. It never occurred to me that I would never play Jansher again, and just as well. If I had known that then, I would never have been able to get through the rest of the evening which I was already starting to dread.

Unfortunately, the humiliation of the match wasn't the only ordeal of the day. There was a post-tournament dinner organised by the sponsors, the Leekes department store in Cardiff. As the two finalists, Jansher and I were expected to attend. It was the last thing I wanted to do but I got ready and went down to the dining room. There were about 50 people there. Everyone was very nice. The sponsors and guests all tried to commiserate with me, but in a way that only made it worse. They told me not to feel bad because I had played well. It wasn't my fault – it was just that Jansher had been brilliant. That was all I got all night; everyone drooling over Jansher's brilliance. It was very frustrating for me. Obviously, I knew that he was a marvellous player, but I had made him look even better because I couldn't perform. But how could I say that to anyone? It was impossible, because it would have looked as if I was making excuses. I didn't want to do that so I had to grin and bear it and agree that yes, Jansher had just been too good on the day.

As soon as the meal was over, I made my way back to the hotel room. I kept trying to understand what had happened. I thought I had probably picked up a virus or something like that. Perhaps if I took it easy for a week or two I would be all right. I went to bed. Normally after a big game like that I would lie awake analysing where the match was won and lost; I would remember my mistakes and make mental notes not to do the same thing again. On this occasion, there was no such analysis. I believed the match had been too much of a one-off disaster to have any relevance for the future. In any case, I had no energy left to be analysing anything. I was exhausted and fell asleep straight away.

I must have slept for 12 hours, but the next morning I still felt drained. I told myself not to worry. I would start feeling better as soon as I had had a good rest. I was wrong. As the adrenaline from the big occasion of the final started to fade, I felt even worse. I couldn't summon the energy or enthusiasm to do anything and was staying in bed all the time. After a big tournament, I would usually take a few days off to relax and recover before starting training again. That's what I had intended to do, but this time it was impossible. I couldn't even think about training. I was sleeping for 13 or 14 hours yet still felt tired.

This went on for a week and then I was due to play Simon Parke in an exhibition match at Ilkeston in Derbyshire. It was the last thing I wanted to do, but I decided to go along just to see how I would shape up. I told Simon how I felt and asked him to go easy on me if he could see I was struggling. My worst fears were confirmed and I found it hard to get around the court. Thankfully, Simon was a good friend and he gave me an easy time. Despite my lethargic performance, I felt better for just having gone out and made the effort. It gave me the confidence to go ahead with a club match I had agreed to play in Holland for Rotterdam.

I knew it was a mistake as soon as I got on the plane. I didn't feel well. I was playing a young Belgian player who I would normally expect to beat quite easily. As it turned out, it was quite a struggle. I managed to win but it was much harder than it should have been. It took too much out of me and did me more harm than good. I went straight to bed when I got home and woke up the next morning to find my glands had swollen up, my throat was sore and my neck was starting to swell. I went to the doctor, who told me it was probably flu and said I could take antibiotics or just rest. I didn't like the idea of taking medication, unless it was unavoidable, so I decided just to take it easy and let the body's natural healing processes take over. I was relieved that I had been given a simple diagnosis which explained away the problem. Lots of people got flu. It would soon be over and I could get back to normal. There was nothing to worry about.

For two weeks I stayed in bed and did nothing. It didn't seem right; things weren't adding up. My glands were no longer enlarged and the swelling on my neck had gone. I no longer had a sore throat and as far as I could see, everything should now be all right. Unfortunately, it wasn't. No matter how much I rested, I still felt worn out. It was disorientating. How long was I supposed to lie there before I started feeling better? Flu didn't behave like this. What else was going on inside me?

As rest didn't seem to be doing me any good, I decided to try some training. Maybe that would kick-start my body back into action. I lasted about five minutes before I had to walk off the court. I couldn't play — there was no energy there at all. All my doubts came hurtling back. This was a lot more than an attack of flu. I was now racked with uncertainty, and that was becoming a problem in itself. As a professional athlete, it had been my business to understand my body. I knew how it worked. I was aware of its nutritional needs. I knew how to train to get the muscles into perfect condition. I could sense when an area wasn't working at full capacity and I knew what to do to put it right. But what was happening now was something different: I didn't understand it, and that was the most frightening thing of all.

I tried to take stock. That had been my approach all my life. Whenever something got in the way I would analyse what was wrong, find the solution then get straight back to the business of playing as soon as possible. That was what I intended to do now, but it was proving more difficult than I thought. There were more tournaments coming up a few weeks later and I also had commitments in Europe. I pulled out of them all. At the time I thought I would probably be out for a month or two while I found out what was wrong and dealt with it. It never occurred to me that I was tackling a problem that would take four years to solve; or that I would have to shed new light on an illness I had suffered as a teenager and had previously thought was isolated and insignificant. How wrong I was about that! Neither did I imagine that I would be forced to reassess my life, my personality and my approach to my profession, and to tame some of the forces that had driven me forward since childhood. It turned out to be the greatest challenge I had ever faced.

# 2.

## MIGHTY MOUSE

My opponent looked at me and seemed puzzled, as if he didn't know whether to be angry or amused. Should he smile and pat me on the head, or frown and give me a hard stare? Looking back on it more than 15 years later, I can understand his confusion. He was an experienced 30-year-old, about six feet tall and probably in the region of 13 stone. I was 12 years old, barely six stones and so small I had to use two hands to hold the racket. We were playing each other in a club match in the Leicestershire Men's League. I had become used to playing against adult opponents but it was nearly always a novelty for them.

As we knocked up before the game, he kept looking back at the rest of my team outside the court to seek some sign that this was a wind-up. Surely they weren't really expecting him to play against this scrawny kid? It was an affront to the man's dignity. He wanted a proper game with someone who could test him. He hadn't given up his evening and travelled all that way to take part in a meaningless walkover. Unfortunately that was exactly what he'd done, but not in the way he thought. Twenty minutes later, it was all over. He lost 3–0 and scarcely got a point.

It was a familiar scenario as my childhood squash career began to gather pace. Most men took their defeat with good grace and were quick to see the funny side. They were usually warm in their congratulations. Some, however, couldn't take the blow to their pride. As soon as they realised they were going to lose, they would try to bully me. They would tower over me whenever they could, shout and swear and argue about points in an effort to intimidate me. Sometimes they would hit the ball as hard as possible, not realising that power without accuracy is pointless.

Thankfully, my opponent this night had behaved himself on court though he still didn't look happy as he wiped the sweat from his forehead

27

and gasped to recover his breath. His pride had obviously been dented but there was worse to come, from his own team-mates. They couldn't resist ribbing him.

'So, Dave, beaten by a kid, eh?' one of them taunted.

A second team-mate tried to soften the blow. 'Well, I suppose he is the British Under-12 champion.'

'Yeah, but he's still a kid though,' said the first man.

'And he can't even hold the racket properly,' said a third.

My opponent gradually regained his composure and a smile broke across his face. He came across to me and pointed a finger at my chest. 'Remind me,' he said, and paused to catch his breath, 'remind me never to play you again.' Then he laughed, shook my hand and asked if I was coming for a pint in the bar.

Perhaps it's not surprising that I showed an early interest in squash. My parents owned a squash club at Kegworth in Leicestershire, which they had built in the '70s when the game was starting to boom. My dad was a keen player and started taking me on court for a gentle knock around when I was about six. My main ambition at that time was to be able to hit the ball hard enough for it to hit the front wall and bounce against the back wall. That was a big thing for me. I wasn't strong enough to hold the heavy wooden rackets with one hand, so I had to use two. The style stuck and was later to become my trademark. I loved the game right from the start and couldn't wait to play. I often used to go on court to practise before going to school. Usually I wanted to practise as soon as I got home from school as well – nothing intense, just half an hour here and there practising my shots or playing matches against friends.

After a few years, I had my first taste of the big time when I got the chance to go on court with Jonah Barrington. It came about because my coach at that time knew him well and occasionally played against him. Jonah was in his late thirties, but was still the British number one and ranked in the world top ten. He agreed to play me for a bit of fun and to give me a lift. It was a fantastic experience. He was, and still is, a legend in the game. I was probably only on court with him for about ten minutes, but he was a great inspiration to me. He seemed intrigued by my two-handed style and was surprised that I was able to use it so effectively. Years later he was to comment that he had never before seen a youngster so advanced in skill and knowledge of the game as I was at that time.

After our brief session on court, Jonah gave me the nickname Mighty Mouse because I was able to hit the ball very hard in spite of my size. The name stuck and was to appear in numerous newspaper headlines over the following few years. Jonah was to become a great help to me throughout my career. Even at that early age, I was determined to try to emulate him. That thought must have been on my mind the following year when I won the British Under-10 championship, beating David Campion in the final. The local paper carried a big article on my victory with the predictable headline of 'Mighty Mouse'. It was one of a series of features called 'Shooting Stars' that they did about youngsters who were aiming for the top. I obviously fitted neatly into that bracket because they quoted me as saying: 'I want to be like Barrington and become British number one. I know there is a long way to go and that it will take a lot of hard work and dedication, but that is my dream.' I was nine at the time.

Like many youngsters, I started playing for my club and entering the regional and national tournaments. It meant several weekends away a year, with my mum and dad ferrying me from venue to venue. This obviously took up a lot of their time, but the competitions became family events and we all enjoyed them. When people read that my family owned a squash club and that I started playing at such a young age they might think my parents tried to force me against my will along a path they had chosen, but nothing could be further from the truth. Both Mum and Dad were very relaxed about me playing the game: they were always supportive, but saw it as nothing more than a source of enjoyment. They never tried to push me in any way and demanded nothing from me other than that I was well-behaved on court.

Sadly, not all parents on the circuit had the same attitude. I remember playing boys who had to endure their fathers constantly shouting at them, trying to spur them on, yet criticising every little mistake they made. There were times when hapless youngsters would be virtually pinned against the wall of the court by irate dads berating them for not playing properly, not getting back to the T, choosing the wrong shots or whatever. 'How many times have I told you?' they would shout. 'You're not concentrating. You're not trying. Think about it! What's the point of us paying for coaching if you're not going to do as you're told?' The father would then turn away in disgust and the boy would be left crestfallen.

There was one lad I remember seeing in an Under-14 tournament who was given a terrible time by his dad. The boy was struggling in his match and the father took it very badly, accusing his son of not trying hard enough. They had a big row when the boy came off court after receiving a real drubbing. The father was so incensed he made him walk the ten miles home just to teach him a lesson. Not surprisingly, such punishments and pep talks rarely resulted in a child performing better. If anything, he would get worse.

My dad used to look on in disbelief when these things happened. Thankfully, he never got angry with me no matter how badly I played. All he asked was that I did my best and behaved myself on court. There could be no arguing with referees. He never criticised me; he just gave advice and encouragement. Dad believed it shouldn't be taken too seriously. Win or lose, it was only a game. Even though I showed early promise, he never talked about me becoming a professional. His attitude seemed to be that if it was meant to happen, then it would. He never tried to get me to do any extra training or anything like that. If anything, he encouraged me to do other sports.

I'm grateful for that because I know I would have resented being shouted at in the way some of my contemporaries were. In the end, for many of those youngsters the constant criticism they were subjected to from their fathers turned out to be counter-productive. Many of them rebelled as they got older and stopped playing altogether. That was quite a loss to the game, because many of them had great talent. No doubt they left with bitter rather than happy memories of what should have been a great childhood experience.

It was certainly a great time for me. Squash is quite a small world in many ways, and I would come across the same faces at most of the major tournaments. I started to make friends with people from all over the country. Many of them are still great friends today. Some didn't quite make it to the top, but enjoyed the game and are still playing just for fun and fitness. Others, like Simon Parke and David Campion, went on to become top-class professionals. We all had ability, obviously, but I think we also had the advantage of having parents who were supportive rather than critical.

We were probably among the first generation of youngsters to enjoy the benefits of the boom in squash in the '80s. Courts were springing up all over the place and the game was getting much more organised thanks to the efforts of national coaches like Edward Poore and Jonah Barrington. I got involved with them when I was nine, after winning the British Under-10 championships, when I got into the England squad and used to go away for coaching at the national squash camps held several times a year at various locations around the country. They were funded mainly by grants from the Sports Council and there was a lot of competition for places.

Jonah Barrington sparked controversy when he introduced national rankings for all levels of the game, even down to the Under-10s. Some people thought this was taking things too seriously at such a young age, and that the intensity of the competition would be bad for us. I can understand what they meant, but I don't think most of the youngsters taking part felt that way. We were all naturally competitive and we just loved playing. The coaches used to complain that, far from forcing us to go on to court, they had a struggle to get us off. That was certainly true. I look back in amazement now at how Simon Parke, David Campion and I would get up at seven so we could get on to the courts before breakfast. I don't think there would be much chance of getting us to do that now, even though we remain passionate about the game.

In my opinion we weren't put under too much pressure, at least not from the coaches. As I have mentioned before, though, some mums and dads could be a problem. I didn't know this at the time, but coaches have since told me about the complaints they constantly get from over-ambitious parents who believe their child hasn't been ranked high enough. They phone up and say little Johnny is much better than so-and-so and should be ranked above him. They point out how hard their boy tries and the number of matches he's won. It doesn't make any difference as the rankings are based purely on results, but that doesn't stop people wanting to sound off. It's crazy and rather sad that they take it so seriously, but it's very much a parent problem rather than a child problem. In this sense, the kids may have more common sense than some of their elders. They're competitive, of course, and they all want to get as high as possible, but they don't get obsessed and unpleasant about it.

The reason for restructuring the youth coaching system in the early eighties was to enable England to create a squad of players who could compete with top nations like Pakistan and Australia. These countries caught their players very young and many coaches, including Barrington and Poore, thought that was the best way forward over here. They were influenced by the progress of a young player called Jahingir Khan who was starting to make a name for himself at that time. He had become the world amateur champion at the age of 15 and went on to win the British Open title, the most prestigious honour in the game, when he was only 17. Jonah Barrington, by contrast, didn't win the first of his six titles until he was over 25. Barrington recognised immediately that Khan was a prodigious talent. He believed, however, that it wasn't just natural ability which had got him to the top so quickly. He had been carefully nurtured since the age of six or seven by some of Pakistan's best coaches. Barrington and Poore realised that if England were to produce champions of a similar standard, they would have to work with players from a similarly tender age.

Both men were aware of the potential pitfalls. The Squash Rackets Association was also monitoring the situation. Its medical adviser, Dr John Williams, watched us very carefully. Having been through the national coaching sessions I can say that I enjoyed them, and I don't think the training did me any harm. The project was certainly successful. Some of the top players of the last ten years were products of those early squash camps. People like Simon Parke, Del Harris and Paul Johnson have all made it into the world's top ten.

But it wasn't all plain sailing for me at the national coaching sessions. I soon started to have problems with a few of the coaches who wanted me to change the way I played. They didn't like my two-handed style and said I wouldn't be able to progress very far beyond the age of 12 if I kept using two hands to grip the racket. They argued that although it might work for tennis, it wouldn't work for squash because the pace was much faster and so there wasn't as much time to adjust between shots. I thought that was nonsense and resented being told to alter the way I played. I thought I was doing fine as I was. But however much I resisted, they were insistent that I needed to change. These coaches sent reports back to my parents pointing out the weaknesses of the two-handed style. They argued that it would limit my reach on court, I wouldn't be able to get the same power and I would put too much stress on my back. My parents were angry about this. They could see that I was upset and not enjoying the game as much. I would come back from the weekend camps feeling quite depressed and complain to them about the attitude of the coaches. One of them used to make me pick up the racket with two fingers and then say: 'There, you can hold the racket with just two fingers, so why do you need to use two hands?' I wasn't impressed. In the end, the insistence of the coaches was counter-productive. The more they tried to make me alter my style, the more I was determined to keep it. I was probably quite stubborn as a child. I wanted to have an equal say in how I played. If it didn't work out, then at least I would know that I had tried in my own way and given it my best shot.

It wasn't that I didn't understand what the coaches were saying. Even at the age of 11 or 12 I could see that there were plusses and minuses to the technique. It undoubtedly limited my reach, and probably put greater strain on my body. On the other hand, I felt it gave me greater control and scope for deception. Using two hands means you need less backswing and so the opponent has less time to assess what you're going to do. I should stress that not all the coaches were urging me to change. People like Jonah Barrington and Mike Hughes were very relaxed about it. Unfortunately, some of the others couldn't let it go and so the battle continued for a year or two. The letters kept getting sent to my parents.

Eventually, my dad decided that he'd had enough. I was becoming more and more miserable and he was worried that I would get disillusioned and not play at all. He wrote a letter back to the coaches saying that enjoyment of the game was the main thing, and urging them to let me carry on playing with two hands if that was what I wanted. Perhaps I'm a little biased, but I think this is very sound advice for all parents and coaches who work with youngsters. If more people had the same attitude, children would have a happier time and more of them would continue playing as they got older. This is an extract from what my dad wrote:

> I was very disappointed to read the coaches have grave doubts about Peter making further progress with his two-handed grip. If that is true, then no doubt you will exclude him from future coaching. We should all realise that Peter will not change his squash style for quite some time and if

we are not careful, he will develop a mental complex that could prove fatal to his squash career.

Surely he must improve, if only by growing taller – thus improving his mobility – and stronger, improving his power. If Peter is coached to improve his use of deception, delayed shots and general fitness, then he will improve whether he plays single-handed, double-handed or a mixture of both.

With regard to his obvious restricted reach, I would suggest that anticipation, speed of reaction, ball control and a squash brain are some of the factors that are more important than reach. If reach were high on the list then I would expect all world squash stars to be over six feet six inches tall.

I would suggest that we encourage Peter to develop his two-handed style and at the same time bring in single-handed shots when necessary, thus helping him to improve all aspects of his game. Sport is littered with excellent junior players who for one reason or another are never heard of as seniors. The chances of Peter becoming a senior star would appear to depend more on determination and good fortune than on some technical aspect of the game.

The last two sentences are particularly telling. I believe many talented youngsters in all sports fall by the wayside and never reach their true potential. There are numerous reasons for this, of course, but I think over-pedantic coaches are a significant factor. Coaching is important but the balance needs to be right. Youngsters need to develop good techniques and they certainly need to gain a good understanding of the game. On the other hand, it's vital that they aren't turned into little machines with each of them being manufactured to play in exactly the same way. Flair and individuality should be allowed to flourish.

The more I think about this, the more strongly I believe that players who do things slightly differently are the ones who stand out from the rest and are often successful. Jonathan Power is a good example. I'm sure he would acknowledge that the way he plays is not what orthodox coaches would call correct. He tends to flick the ball and uses a short backswing.

That would once have been considered technically wrong, yet it is one of the things that makes him such a difficult opponent because it is so deceptive. If he had been brought up in a strict coaching regime, he may have had a lot of that knocked out of him. Fortunately that didn't happen, so he was able to develop into one of the best and most charismatic players on the circuit, showing that people can be that bit different and still come through and excel.

As a boy I was sure I could do well too, if I were allowed to develop my own style. Thankfully, the coaches stopped pressurising me after my dad wrote to them and I was able to start enjoying the game a lot more. I remained a little wary for a long time afterwards, however. For a few years I hardly had any coaching at all because I was worried that they would start trying to make me change again. I wanted to get to the top even at that early age, but I was sure I could do it my own way. I could see that I was developing and getting better – I was winning most of my matches – so what was the point in changing to a style that could make me worse? This meant I was left to my own devices to a certain extent. I couldn't get coaching in the technicalities of using two hands because no one had any experience of it. I had to work it out for myself.

When I was at the national coaching sessions, I restricted myself to learning as much as possible about tactics, where to place the ball and when to go for certain types of shots. That kind of match-play advice came to represent the main thing that coaches had to offer me and I gratefully took on board everything they had to say. But as for my style, I was determined to carry on as I was. Perhaps I was just being stubborn, but I think it's quite likely that if I had been persuaded to change then I might not have gone on to become a professional. As I got older, the coaches came to accept my approach and my relationship with them improved. I began to work on one-handed shots, but only to get me out of trouble as a last resort when the ball was placed out of my reach or came at an unexpected pace.

Squash wasn't my only game when I was young. I played football at school, although I wasn't all that good. I also enjoyed athletics and golf. I managed to get into the Leicestershire county tennis squad, which suggests that racket sports were my main strength. It wasn't long before squash came to dominate, however, and I gave up playing tennis.

I was quite shy at school. Squash helped to build my confidence because I was good at it. It suited my competitive nature and I liked the fact that it was stimulating mentally as well as physically. You had to put a lot of thought into outwitting your opponent and moving him out of position. Squash began to play a very important role in my life. It was a way of expressing myself, and it gave me a great deal. I'm sure that sport can be a very positive force for all youngsters.

By the time I was 12, I was competing regularly in the Leicestershire men's league. I managed to get the better of most of my older opponents but no matter how hard I tried there was one person who always seemed to beat me: my dad. All kids are desperate to upstage their parents and I was no exception. Dad hadn't started playing squash until he was in his 30s but he was very enthusiastic and became a good county player. Like many people who have a lot of natural ability but haven't had any coaching he developed his own style, which was awkward to play against. He didn't hit the ball very hard. It was all slow lobs and then tight drop shots. It was effective, and I couldn't get the better of him. There was also a psychological aspect to it, of course. As a child, you get used to seeing your dad as a tower of strength and it can be hard to imagine that you could ever beat him. Consequently, there was a period when I was losing to him even though I had surpassed him and should have been getting some convincing victories. I could beat several players who could beat him, but I couldn't do it myself.

Nevertheless, after several defeats I was getting to a stage where I thought I could get my first victory. My chance came when I was promoted into the same league as him at our local club. It was just the ordinary box league that all squash players will recognise, but to me it was a great opportunity to beat him in a full competitive match. I was very serious about it and went into it full of confidence. Sadly, that confidence was misplaced. He beat me quite easily. I don't think I've ever been so upset about losing a squash match, before or since. I brooded over it for days. Thinking you should be able to beat your dad and then losing to him amounts to a disaster when you're 12. I think I was also a bit annoyed that he had tried to beat me so convincingly. Perhaps it was his way of making sure I didn't get too cocky, or perhaps he wanted to show me that I still had a long way to go.

Dad didn't say anything to me immediately after my defeat. He obviously decided to give me a few hours to calm down. After a while, though, the inevitable ribbing started. He was in his forties at that time, so he kept saying how surprising it was that an old man like him could beat a fit young lad like me. I wasn't in much of a mood for joking to begin with but I soon saw the funny side of it. I think he was keen to make sure I didn't take things too seriously, which was a good thing. I eventually cheered up but I didn't forget my annoyance at losing. It spurred me on. I began to practise even harder and then I beat him a few months later. That was it. Dad never beat me again. It may be significant, however, that I remember that defeat much more vividly than I remember the following victory. I hated losing, even at that young age. I was always prepared to work hard to improve. I don't know where that attitude came from. No one put any pressure on me, yet somehow I developed an overwhelming desire to succeed. It must have been part of my make-up.

Thankfully, I was winning far more games than I was losing and the game was even starting to take me abroad occasionally. When I was 12, I became the Swiss Under-14 champion. Simon Parke was also there competing. It was good to win, but the trip remains in my memory for a very different reason. It was our first encounter with girls. We were staying in an old army barracks with male and female quarters. Simon and I were a lot less shy then than we are now and I remember us running into the female dormitories shouting and showing off in front of some Swedish girls. We even jumped on their beds. They were probably only about 17 but to us they seemed beautiful, sophisticated women of the world. They treated us like the little boys we were but seemed quite taken with us all the same. They made a fuss of us in an older sister sort of way and we became good friends for the week. Looking back, it was probably one of our more successful exploits with women. We certainly wouldn't have the nerve to go running through the female dormitories now!

Shortly after returning from Switzerland, I became the England number one at Under-14 level and went on to win the British Under-14 title. Those were two big milestones for me. No matter how successful I was, however, the arguments about my two-handed style continued. Having finally convinced my coaches to let me continue as I wanted I then had to explain it away to reporters and other well-meaning but ill-advised squash enthusiasts who thought I should change. The debate about my style often overshadowed the fact that I had just won a tournament, even something as significant as a British title. I was always being asked if it wouldn't be a good idea to change to playing one-handed as I would almost certainly get better results. I would think to myself: 'But I've just become British champion. What better result could there be than that?'

Jonah Barrington helped me at this stage by publicly backing me. On the eve of the British Open Under-14 championships, he dismissed criticism of my style by telling the press that I was one of the brightest prospects in the country. 'As long as he continues to develop I am not going to interfere with his natural grip. No matter how unnatural it looks to others.' It was good to get a public seal of approval from the great man. His support didn't stop the criticism, but it helped. It certainly made me feel better about it.

I also got a lot of support from another top coach, Malcolm Willstrop, who has developed something of a squash dynasty. He's the stepdad of David Campion and the father of James Willstrop who became British junior champion and is now making a name for himself on the professional circuit. I used to attend Malcolm's squash camps in the school holidays and I really enjoyed them. Sometimes I would be there for up to five weeks during the summer. Like Jonah, he was very relaxed about my two-handed style. He guided me through a lot of the finer points of the game but never bothered about my style. That meant a lot to me.

---

Throughout my childhood, I had been attending the local schools and was very happy with them. Then, when I was about 15, I got the chance to go to the exclusive Millfield School in Somerset. It was very expensive but it had a strong sporting tradition and great facilities, with several squash courts and indoor tennis courts, as well as numerous playing fields covering all sorts of sports. The set-up was probably better than that of many universities. The main attraction for me, however, was that Jonah Barrington worked there as squash coach. I thought it would help me develop as a player and my parents agreed to let me go.

I arrived with great hopes but it turned out to be the worst period of my childhood. It wasn't me at all – a real culture shock. I had been used to going to my local comprehensive school at Castle Donington in Leicestershire. It was a good school; very modern, and very relaxed in its attitudes. Millfield, by contrast, was one of the country's great public schools and was steeped in a much more conformist tradition. To be fair, it was probably one of the more enlightened of our fee-paying schools but to me, coming from my very relaxed background, it all seemed very regimented. It had a prefect system in which the older kids were able to tell the younger ones what to do. Shortly after I arrived, one of the prefects made me do some housework for him. He was hovering over me all the time as I swept up. He kept pointing out little bits that I had missed, or that he said I had missed. I hated it. Everyone had chores to do and I didn't mind that. It was the way it was done, with prefects constantly watching and obviously revelling in the power they had.

I didn't like the school system either. I found the whole lifestyle very restrictive. I was assigned things constantly and given very little free time. The whole day was mapped out for me and everywhere I turned there were people telling what I could and couldn't do. It was a little bit like the time when I was being pressurised by the coaches who wanted me to change the way I played. I rebelled against it. There was something about me that resented being told what to do.

I became very unsettled. The people there weren't really my types either. They were very wealthy and perhaps a bit spoilt; they had all the latest gadgetry. When I arrived, I brought a cassette player with me. As soon as the others saw it, they started taking the mickey because they had the very latest CD players, which at that time were very expensive and way beyond the reach of most kids. I wouldn't have minded the normal ribbing and banter you inevitably get in all groups of people, but I found their assumption of superiority based purely on their parents' wealth to be distasteful and a bit pathetic. It was an attitude that came out even more in the way they spoke about the local kids in the area. They were very disparaging about their backgrounds and called them insulting names. This made things awkward for me. When you're young, there is always pressure on you to behave like your peers and fit in with the crowd. Everybody wants to belong rather than be an outsider. It would have been easy to go along with their snobbish attitude as a way of blending in, but it just wasn't me. It left me feeling a bit isolated.

The only good thing about the place for me was Jonah Barrington. He helped me a lot but in spite of his efforts, my game went backwards while

I was at Millfield because I was so unhappy. My time there was very lonely and I couldn't wait to get away. It wasn't being away from home that bothered me: I had spent lots of time away from my parents at various squash camps. The problem was the ethos of the place and the attitudes of so many of the people around me. I stuck it out at first, because I had heard that many people don't like boarding school to begin with but change their minds after a while when they've had a chance to get used to it. I'm afraid I never came to terms with it. I stayed for a year and then returned home. It wasn't that there was anything wrong with Millfield specifically, it was more the boarding school approach in general. It just wasn't for me.

I went back to my local school but because of my unhappy time at Millfield, I was a year behind and ended up doing my GCSEs at the same time as Simon Parke. He used to tease me about being a bit fuzzy-headed and I don't think he expected me to do all that well in my exams. Even now, he thinks I'm a strange character; clumsy and with a poor short-term memory. He concedes that when people get to know me they realise that I'm okay. It's just that I sometimes come across as a bit absent-minded and other-worldly. I don't think I'm like that at all, but as I admit to doing things like going away for the weekend leaving my door wide open, I can't really argue.

I was at Simon's house in Knaresborough on the day of the exam results. Simon phoned his school and found that he'd got five GCSEs and one O Level, a result he was pleased with. Then it was my turn. Simon says he remembers I was on the phone looking anxious when suddenly a big smile lit up my face. I put the phone down and told him I had got two As and seven Bs. He looked totally dumbfounded. Then he said: 'Are you sure you've got the right results?' It wasn't quite the vote of confidence I was looking for, but he just couldn't quite take it in. 'Are you sure they're not someone else's results?' he insisted, still shaking his head. The worst of it was that everyone else reacted in much the same way.

I didn't mind. Things were now going well on all fronts. My game had recovered dramatically after leaving Millfield and I was now the British Under-16 champion. It was crunch time for deciding what I was going to do next. I wanted to turn professional but knew that it might be more sensible to stay on at school and take A Levels. After all, many promising youngsters don't make it as professionals. There was never any serious debate in my mind, however. I wanted to play and that was that. My parents didn't try to talk me out of it. They knew that if they did force me to stay on at school I probably wouldn't work very hard anyway, so it would be pointless. I decided to take the plunge and it was an incredibly exciting feeling. The plan was to try it for a year and see how it went. If I was a total disaster then I could always go back to doing my A Levels.

That, at least, is what I told myself. In reality, however, I had no intention of failing. I was determined to succeed no matter how hard it would be. I knew it would take a lot more than just talent. To get to the top I would have to be focused, dedicated and show an irrepressible will to win. I knew I had those qualities in abundance. They had made me one of the most outstanding players in my age group and I was confident they could take me right to the top.

# 3.
## THE NEW KID ON THE BLOCK

Stepping up to professional level was entering a new world. The attitude and mindset were far more hostile than anything I had experienced on the amateur circuit. The top players weren't prepared to give you an inch; not a word of encouragement and certainly no advice. They would look at your game and very quickly work out how to play you. They would then wipe the floor with you in a match. Afterwards they would make no comment about the game or how they had exploited your weaknesses. They wouldn't give you a clue about anything.

The Australian Chris Dittmar was especially intimidating. He took no prisoners at all. He was a big guy, and he liked to come across as frightening. Chris wouldn't give anything away on court, and after the game he wouldn't let you get to know him very well. It was all part of his act. He probably felt that it might make it harder for you to play him. I got on all right with him, but we weren't friends. I quickly discovered that this was the way things were at the top level in the professional game at that time. The top players didn't socialise with the younger ones as they did lower down the ranks. It was far removed from the family atmosphere of the weekend amateur events I had been used to as a youngster.

Perhaps it was a cross-cultural thing – the leading two players, Jahingir and Jansher Khan, were from Pakistan. The linguistic and cultural differences meant they didn't mix with players from other countries very much. The English and Australians shared the same language, but were divided by an intense rivalry. People like Chris Dittmar and Rodney Martin were among the best players of the day. They saw people like me and Simon Parke as young upstarts who were trying to challenge their supremacy, and were very keen to put us in our place. A squash court is quite small so you're always very close physically to your opponent. It's a little like being in a boxing ring. Players will often bump into each other and it's possible for one to impose himself on the other and come across as intimidating. Sometimes a young player needs to be very mentally strong to cope with this.

Martin, Dittmar and the other top pros wanted not only to beat us; they wanted their victories to be as easy as possible, so they took every opportunity to grind us into the dust. They thought that if they could do this while we were still young and green then it would make it harder for us to beat them in the future when we started to mature. This can happen in squash, and may affect a player's career. An experienced pro can get such a psychological advantage over a youngster that the youngster never recovers. He finds he still can't beat the older guy years later when really he should be able to do so easily. I was determined not to let that happen to me. In fact, I liked the attitude of the top players because at least you knew where you stood with them. I didn't want them to mess about with me. I wanted them to give me their best game, even if it meant I took a few drubbings at their hands. I didn't mind. I was learning all the time and I knew the pain of defeat would make the pleasure of victory all the sweeter when it came.

In many ways those first few years were the best and most exciting of my career. I was just like any youngster starting his first job after leaving school. I wasn't sure about things and had to learn as I went along. I wasn't on my own, of course. All across the world there were young players just like me taking their first steps on the professional circuit. I think I knew even then that only a handful of the hundreds of young hopefuls would make it to the top. Most would fall by the wayside for all sorts of reasons. They might not have quite enough ability. Even if they did they might struggle with injuries, or perhaps they might find it hard to cope with the lifestyle and the travelling. Finance would be another problem. It's hard in the early days to earn enough money to keep going. I knew all about the potential pitfalls, but nothing could put me off. It seemed very glamorous to be travelling the country to compete against players I had been paying money to see only a few months earlier. Every game I played was special and I couldn't wait for the next tournament to come around. It was also a time of very little pressure because, as the newcomer, you aren't really expected to beat any of the seasoned pros and yet you're looking for scalps everywhere.

Simon and I had our first major success at the Lee-on-the-Solent Men's Open in 1988. It was hardly the biggest tournament in the world, but it still attracted several players who were in the top ten in England. We were rank outsiders and so were drawn to play the two favourites in the first round. I had the number two seed Andrew Danzie and Simon was up against Mark Cairns who was seeded number one. They were both long-established England internationals and we were regarded as brash young imposters. This was brought home to Simon when he overheard a conversation between a spectator and Mark Cairns. The fan said something like: 'I see you're drawn against Simon Parke. He's a decent young prospect. He should give you a good game.'

Cairns was very dismissive and replied: 'You must be joking. I'll be too strong for him. I'll soon sort him out. He's just a young muppet.'

That wasn't a wise thing to say. Simon plays like a man possessed at the best of times but that just fired him up even more. He went on court determined to make Cairns eat his words. He was brilliant and won 3–0. He was only 16 at the time. It was his first win over someone who was older, stronger and a seasoned professional. I chalked up a similar first by beating Andrew Danzie. Having tasted victory we got a momentum going and we both went all the way, meeting in the final. I won 3–1 in a very tough game. It was a huge tournament for us, because we proved to ourselves that we could perform against established pros. It gave us confidence knowing we belonged in that circle. We learnt a great deal from the experience, but I think the more established players also learnt a thing or two as well – not to underestimate us and, more importantly, not to call Simon Parke a muppet!

After my success at Lee-on-the-Solent, I was keen to start competing in the bigger tournaments. It was very hard to break through, though. The odds were stacked against the newcomer. The established pros in the top 24 had all the advantages: they didn't have to qualify for the major tournaments, so they could start in the first round proper, fresh and in perfect shape. We had to wade through various qualifying rounds; the lower down the rankings you were, the more qualifying matches you had to play. This could be an exhausting ordeal. The established pros were also able to stay in comfortable hotels paid for by the tournament organisers, while those of us outside the magic 24 had to find our own accommodation and as we weren't earning much money, it was usually pretty basic.

I remember competing in a tournament at Altdorf in Germany when I was 18. I was beginning to make a bit of progress, but was still outside the world top 250. It meant that in the qualifiers I had to play three matches on the same day. I played one at 4 p.m. which I won 3–0, then another at 7 p.m. when I came through 3–1, then another at ten that evening when the score was 3–2. I couldn't afford expensive hotel bills so I had to sleep on the floor at the home of one of the tournament staff. We often had to impose on people's goodwill in that way. Then I had to be back on court at ten the next morning to play the next round. I lost, which is hardly surprising after the efforts of the day before. If I had managed to win, I would have had to play again that night and then twice the next day.

There simply isn't enough money in the game to enable tournament organisers to help players trying to qualify. This means that young hopefuls can be excluded from big events because they can't afford to get there. For example, if you want to compete in the Hong Kong Open, it means paying around £700 air fare so that you can fly out about a week before the top players to compete in the qualifying rounds. When you get there, your hotel bill and other expenses might come to another thousand pounds. If you're successful and fight your way through to the main draw, then you might be all right: the tournament sponsors will then provide hotel accommodation. If you get through a few rounds, perhaps to the quarter-finals, then you might start to make a bit of a profit, perhaps a thousand pounds if you're really lucky. On the other hand, if you lose in the qualifying rounds you don't earn a penny. You could easily find yourself losing a couple of thousand pounds on the journey. What's more, you don't earn any ranking points so the whole trip has been an expensive waste of time. It's little wonder that many talented players fall by the wayside because they simply can't afford to keep going.

The courts and facilities were often very poor at that level. I played in a tournament in Germany where they hadn't sealed the floor of the court properly, so it became wet and very slippery. We were sliding all over the place. We often met similar problems in places like Pakistan, India and

Malaysia. The main tournament courts in those countries would be fine, but in the qualifying rounds, and even in the early stages of the main tournaments, you were often placed on back courts which were substandard. The walls were sometimes crooked and it wasn't uncommon to find two or three floorboards askew. The ball would go bouncing in all directions.

Sometimes the state of the court could lead to farcical situations, even in the later stages of a tournament. I remember playing Simon in the final of the Italian Open. It was on an outdoor court and unfortunately there had been a heavy downpour of rain. They tried to sweep it clean and dry, but weren't having much luck. Eventually we had to go ahead and make a game of it. After four or five points, however, it became clear that it was simply impossible to play properly. We were both slipping around all over the place. The organisers agreed to declare the match void and play it the following day on an indoor court. That was fine, except the game was being televised live and the producers wanted something to show. Simon and I had to go back on court and play out a mock final for the benefit of the television audience. We were still slipping about so goodness knows what they made of it. Simon won the TV match but I reversed the result the next day to take the title. It must be the only action replay in history in which the result changed!

The worst problem, however, was when there was no air conditioning. This wasn't so bad in the evenings, but often the tournament timetable meant you had to play in the midday sun. Within 20 minutes your head would feel as though it was boiling. After about a game and a half, you would be ready to explode. You might go off court to try to get some fresh air, but it would be so humid you wouldn't be able to breathe properly. Then you would look across at your opponent, and if he was a local player he'd be smiling and looking fine because he was used to the conditions.

Those early days were very much an extension of our amateur days and it took us quite a while to develop a fully professional attitude. I was still mixing with the players I had been brought up with; people like Simon, David Campion and Del Harris. We had all enjoyed a lot of back-up as juniors from the Squash Rackets Association and coaches like Jonah Barrington. But as soon as we turned professional, we were on our own. Nowadays, the lottery puts money in to help young players, so there are coaches and teams of sports scientists to offer much-needed help. In those days, there was nothing. Jonah said at the time that the lack of proper support was damaging to our progress and when I look back, I see what he meant. We weren't too well organised and created all sorts of problems for ourselves with our typically teenage approach. Sometimes we would miss the chance to play in tournaments because we would forget to get the application forms in before the closing date.

One year, Simon and I decided to play a tournament in Germany and made a special effort to make sure we entered on time. We were about to fly out and were feeling very pleased with ourselves for our organisational skills when we realised we'd booked flights to the wrong country. The tournament was at Altdorf in Germany, but we'd booked to go to Altdorf in Switzerland! We had to make a nine-hour rail journey to get to the right place. And to cap it all, we had to sleep on someone's floor when we got there. We didn't win, but we got through the first few rounds so it wasn't a complete disaster. In spite of everything, we enjoyed the trip and several others like them.

---

I did reasonably well in my first two years. Then I suffered a big setback. It was in May 1989, and I had just turned 18. I had recently returned from a tournament in Austria when I woke up one morning with a headache and a sore throat. My glands started to swell up, and I felt tired. I thought it was tonsillitis, a condition I had suffered from every year throughout my teens, so I didn't worry too much about it. I didn't expect it to last long, but after a few weeks I still wasn't feeling any better. Tonsillitis would have usually run its course by then, so I went to see my doctor. He did some blood tests and told me I had glandular fever. I had no idea how I caught it but it really knocked me out. I was advised not to play or train but there was no question of that anyway. I felt too tired and drained to do anything.

The illness came just at the wrong time for me. I was about to play in my first World Open championships in Malaysia, but had to pull out. I also missed out on my first chance to play for England in the world team championships. It was very disappointing. Simon Parke, David Campion and Del Harris went off to represent their country, but I had to stay at home in bed. I remember lying there wishing I could be playing and training. The glandular fever stopped me doing anything. For the first two weeks I was very ill and after that I felt tired all the time. My glands kept swelling up and then returning to normal, before swelling up again. Fortunately it was the end of the season, so I didn't miss out on too many tournaments, but it meant I couldn't do any training over the summer.

After about four months, I was starting to feel stronger and went back for more blood tests. I was told the glandular fever had cleared up – I was clear to start training. Although I still didn't feel 100 per cent, I was eager to get on with things; it had been very frustrating to be out. At that age, you want to be playing and training all the time. Four months off the circuit seems like an eternity. I felt I had a lot of catching up to do. Looking back, I probably should have waited longer before starting to push myself really hard, but at the time I didn't know any better.

For the first few months I was playing even though I still didn't feel quite right. I couldn't put my finger on what was wrong, but I knew I wasn't the same as before. It didn't seem to matter too much, though – I eventually regained my strength and felt I was back to normal. I forgot all about the glandular fever. Apart from the interruption to my progress, I didn't see it as having any long-term significance. Years later, events were to prove me wrong.

At the time, however, all I could think of was returning to work. Thankfully, I soon got back into my stride and notched up my first big titles, winning the world Under-19 and Under-23 championships within ten days of each other. I was 18 at the time. I beat Simon Parke in the Under-19 final, and Colin Keith in the Under-23s. It was now the end of 1989. I had been a professional for just over two years. I was ranked at number 11 in England and had a world ranking of 80. I was reasonably pleased with that, but was looking to make a big improvement over the following year. I set myself the target of breaking into the England top ten and the world top 40 by the following September. It would be a difficult task, but my two victories in the Under-19 and Under-23 tournaments were a big turning point and gave me lots of confidence.

I was working hard, but overall it was an easygoing time. Simon and I were trying to do well, of course, but we still looked on things in a lighthearted way and tried to enjoy ourselves. Unfortunately, that approach got us into big trouble with Jonah Barrington during the European team championships in 1991. I was playing for England alongside Simon, Del Harris and David Campion. Jonah was the coach. The tournament was being held in Spain. Although Jonah demanded total dedication during the matches and training, he let us go our own way during the evenings. For us that meant going straight out to the clubs to relax and enjoy the nightlife, just like any other group of lads at the time. We were drinking, but not excessively. The main problem was that we would stay out until the early hours of the morning and often got only a few hours' sleep before having to go out on court and compete.

We were still winning but not as easily as we should have been, considering the standard of the players we were competing against. Jonah was angry and things came to a head when I got to 2–2 against a player I should have beaten 3–0. Before the start of the fifth game, Jonah got us all together and gave us a real roasting, telling us that we were all unprofessional and we'd never get anywhere if we carried on like that. He seemed to take it out on me more than the others, possibly because I was the one most obviously not coming up to my usual standard. I went back on court and managed to complete a 3–2 win. The others won as well, so we ended up with a 5–0 victory despite our night-time activities. However, we still left the tournament with Jonah's words ringing in our ears. He was right, of course, and he had an effect on us. Jonah has quite a temper, and he's not the kind of person you ignore. We won the tournament, but we probably only got away with it because we were so young and the opposition wasn't that strong. There was no way we could be successful if we carried on that way. We were all a little more careful after that.

Simon and I started to be seen as two of the fittest and most determined young players on the circuit. This was illustrated when we met in the Dutch Open in 1990. We had got in to the top five in England but were still very much the young pretenders, particularly on the world stage. Our match in Holland turned out to be a classic physical battle. Neither of us was prepared to give an inch and we slugged it out like street fighters for over two hours. Both Simon and I were very quick, and were each able to put the other under pressure. There were very few mistakes or unforced errors. It went to five sets, with me just shading it in what was a brutal war of attrition. I felt strong and fit – as if I could fight on forever. It was wonderful to take part in such a battle. The spectators were captivated by it. The Welsh international Aidan Davies, who went on to win the tournament, said it was the hardest game of squash he had ever seen. It was another landmark in our developing careers and made people realise how determined we were. No one could expect to beat us without us putting up a fight.

We were far from being the finished article, however, as was made painfully clear to me when I played my first matches against established world-class opponents Chris Dittmar and Chris Robertson. I met Dittmar in the British Open and was excited because he had been one of my boyhood heroes. I had watched him play several times and studied videos of him. I knew he was way above me but with that strange blind confidence of youth, I half-believed I might beat him. He soon blew away any such illusions. Within a few rallies, it became clear that he was in a different league from me then. His pace, power and accuracy were just too much for me to handle. I was sent scampering all over the court trying to retrieve his shots. I had never before tired so quickly on a squash court. Within just ten minutes, I was starting to feel exhausted and felt I was one of the most unfit players there had ever been. I was struggling to breathe, and my legs were burning.

One of the things that struck me most at the time was how seriously Dittmar was taking the game. He was beating me so easily it was almost embarrassing, yet he remained totally focused. There was no way he was going to mess about with me; he was even taking advice from his coach in between games. He wanted to play even better. It made me realise how professional Dittmar was. He probably realised he might have to play me several times in the future and wanted to set a precedent by beating me as easily as possible.

As if the drubbing by Dittmar wasn't enough, I then came up against Chris Robertson in the early rounds of the Kiel Open in Germany. Chris was another tough and highly talented Australian who had no compunction about beating young hopefuls. I gave the match everything I had, but he beat me easily by three games to nil. As with Dittmar, the pace was too fast for me. I was run ragged. I realised that although I had made rapid progress over the previous two years, there was a massive difference between them and me at that point. I had a lot of work to do.

One of the most noticeable things about both Dittmar and Robertson was how quick they were to exploit my two-handed style. They worked out straight away where its weaknesses lay – they kept putting the ball tight into the forehand corner because it exposed my lack of reach. They also used a lot of high lobs to my forehand for the same reason. Both had the tactical awareness to see my limitations and the skill to expose them. It was very impressive. My two main qualities as a player, my fitness and mental strength, were of little help against Dittmar and Robertson because they were able to outplay me so easily. It gave me a lot to think about, but I wasn't too despondent. I realised that I could learn a lot from what had happened. I would have to improve my one-handed play so that I could get out of trouble when necessary. I also had to improve my overall game so that I wouldn't be put under pressure in the first place.

Playing Dittmar and Robertson helped to sharpen me up, and I made rapid progress through 1990. By the following October I had surpassed the targets I'd set for myself; I had become the England number 2 and jumped to number 33 in the world. My health was still causing me occasional problems, however. It was nothing major and I certainly didn't think anything of it at the time. But looking back, I can see that I seemed to get colds and sniffles much more than most people. It was as if I was just that little bit more prone to illness. Every year there would be a week or two when I didn't feel quite right. It was nothing definite and I was even sometimes uncertain as to whether anything was wrong. If I did suspect anything, I would put it to the back of my mind because I wanted to push on. Before long, I would get back to normal and forget all about it.

---

In 1990 I had to pull out of the US Open because of flu. It wasn't a big deal, but it was disappointing to miss such a big tournament. Thankfully, I was only confined to bed for five days. I didn't want to lie around any longer than I had to, because I wanted to be ready to compete in the qualifying rounds of the Canadian Open. I was in two minds about whether or not I was fit enough to play, but I decided to go for it. It was the right decision. I gained the two biggest wins of my career so far and gave Chris Robertson a major scare.

I got through the qualifying rounds okay, and then came up against Mir Zaman Gul. He was ranked seventh in the world, and was expected to beat me easily. I didn't expect to win but I knew I was getting closer and closer to the top players. I was determined to go out and give it everything I had. As always, I wanted to pick up at least a game or two and make it as difficult as possible for Mir. In the end, I surpassed my wildest expectations. I felt very strong on court and the extra pace and quality that you always find with a top-class opponent didn't bother me at all. I won in straight sets. I was so delighted you would think I had won the tournament, rather than just the first round! It was satisfying to win, of course. But it was also reassuring to know that I could come through when the opportunity presented itself. I had been able to hold my nerve when I realised that victory was possible and I got to match ball. I didn't freeze or bottle it, as so often happens with young sports players when suddenly confronted with the prospect of winning at the top level.

It was a fantastic feeling but I couldn't savour it for long because there was an even bigger challenge to come. My opponent in the second round was my England team-mate Del Harris, who like me had suffered a roasting from Jonah that day in Spain. He was and still is a superb player who became British number one when he was only 18. For about three years afterwards he was unbeaten in England. Not only that, but he had a string of victories against me dating from our time as juniors. Del was a couple of years older than me, and had been about a foot taller when we were children. The difference in age and size gave him an advantage I hadn't been able to overcome and I had never beaten him. Nevertheless, I fancied my chances as I prepared to play him. We were both adults now: he no longer towered over me and I was brimming with confidence having beaten Mir Zaman Gul.

In the end, I got another straight sets victory. I was so pleased I can still remember the score. It was 15–10, 15–8, 15–10. I was walking on air when I came off court, already looking forward to future encounters. Having beaten Del once I was determined to go on beating him. I was confident I could replace him as the British number one.

In the meantime, however, there was a more pressing matter. In the third round I was up against Chris Robertson, the man who had so clinically taught me the difference in standard between top professionals and young hopefuls when I played him the year before. I wasn't nearly as confident of winning as I had been in the previous two matches, but I was determined to do better than the humiliating drubbing I had suffered in our previous match. I thought I could make him fight all the way, take several points and maybe even a game.

It would be like a fairytale to be able to say that I beat him, but it wasn't to be. I got a victory of sorts, though, in surpassing my expectations by taking him all the way to the end. He beat me, but at 3–2 it was uncomfortably close for him. Having got so near, I was a little disappointed but, being realistic, I knew that I had played out of my skin and had done incredibly well. He still had too much for me to cope with but I had served notice that I was a force to be reckoned with by taking two games off him. The gap between us had narrowed considerably and there was every chance I would go one better the next time. I think I was probably looking forward to our next meeting a lot more than he was.

That run in the Canadian Open really made people take notice of me. The press suddenly showed an interest and wanted my reaction to the game against Robertson. I said I was a bit surprised to have done so well but had always thought I could pull off a victory against Del, and that I fancied my chances against anyone outside the top five. I suppose that was a big statement for a 19-year-old, but it was a mark of my growing confidence. I really thought I could get to the top.

I was pleased to see that some of the older pros agreed with me. The *Sunday Telegraph* carried a large article on my progress over the previous year and asked the New Zealand star Ross Norman to assess my potential. He was quoted as saying: 'Six months at that age can make an incredible difference. He's stronger, he's fitter, he's more consistent, he drives better and he understands the game more. He not only beat Harris, he beat him comprehensively. Mir and Del played as well as Marshall let them. He relentlessly pressured Del into making mistakes and the winners he hit far outweighed anything Del had to offer.' Of course, there had to be the inevitable questions raised about my two-handed style. Thankfully, Norman was positive. 'He's confounded everyone. Critics said he's going to do his back in, he's going to get injuries, you can't hit a ball like that, but he's doing it.' It made satisfying reading considering all the criticism my two-handed style had received over the years.

During those first few years I worked hard to become a good professional, although I suppose there was still the air of an amateur about me off the court. I had no agent or manager. I just did the best I could and learnt it all as I went along. My first sponsorship deal was negotiated by Simon Parke's father. He'd been helping Simon and offered to help me as well. The terms were good, so I signed. It didn't strike me as strange at the time, although it might seem very laid-back to some people now. I didn't particularly mind how much money I made as long as it was enough to survive on.

In 1991, I set off to compete in the World Open in Adelaide. I had never been to Australia before and was determined to make the most of it. That was a great time for me, although the flight out there was a bit embarrassing: I went through check-in at Heathrow with Simon Parke without any trouble, but then I stopped to make a phone call. My passport was still in my hand so I placed it on top of the coin box as I picked up the receiver. I made the call and then, in my absent-minded way, walked off forgetting all about the passport. Of course, they wouldn't let me onto the plane without it. I had no idea what I had done with it, and this prompted a big panic. The airline people tried to help me find it and, of course, I was getting more and more embarrassed as I tried to remember where I had left it. We were already cutting it fine and the minutes began to tick away without any sign of the passport.

Take-off time approached, but as my bags had already been placed on the plane they couldn't leave without me. For obvious security reasons, people aren't allowed to put bags on a plane unless they go on the flight themselves. It would have been a major task to unload my baggage and I think the aircraft staff were also a bit worried that they had perhaps forgotten to return my passport at check-in and so may have been partly responsible. Whatever the reason, they continued to wait several minutes past the set take-off time.

A stewardess eventually found the passport where I had left it on the phone. She handed it over, and I made my way down the aisle while the pilot announced that they had eventually sorted out the person who was holding everyone up. It was like running the gauntlet with people giving me dirty looks and mumbling abuse. There was worse to come. As I sat down hoping to dissolve anonymously into my seat, the pilot came up and said we would now have to wait another hour to take off because he had missed his slot. It would cost the airline thousands of pounds to pay for another one. I was 20 years old, but was made to feel like a naughty schoolboy. The flight to Australia is long enough as it is, but that incident made it seem ten times longer. In the confined space of the plane, there was no escape from the disapproving looks of the other passengers.

It wasn't the best of starts to a world open but I soon perked up when I arrived in Australia. We had travelled out three weeks before the start of the tournament to acclimatise, sample the country and see how squash was organised in Australia. We were staying at the Australian Institute of Sport, the country's main centre for squash, based in Brisbane. All the top Australian players trained there including Brett and Rodney Martin, their sister Michelle, Sarah Fitzgerald, Chris Dittmar, Rodney Eyles and many more. They had all come through the institute as juniors, which is one of the reasons they developed so well and so fast. We quickly realised what we'd been missing back home in England in terms of back-up and support. The whole set-up was designed to provide squash players with everything they needed both on and off the court. The institute had houses that the players were free to use whenever they wanted. There were even domestic staff to cook and clean for them. They also had sports scientists to work out gym programmes, medical back-up, doctors, physiotherapists. Everything.

All this gave the Australian players a tremendous advantage over us and probably most other players in the world. They could all go there and work together, swap ideas and have regular practice matches against players of their own standard. They also had the extra bonus of being able to call on Geoff Hunt for help and advice; the eight times British Open winner worked there as a coach and was able to pass on the benefit of his great experience. There would be four or five courts going at the same time. Hunt would watch the different matches and then go on court to give the players pointers about their game. We felt we were very much the poor relations. There was no such centre in England. We were all far more isolated and had to make our own arrangements: this often meant travelling across the country just to get practice matches against someone of a similar standard.

The institute management made us very welcome and allowed us to stay in one of their houses. We spent two great weeks training with the Australians and playing regular practice matches with them. It was a fantastic experience. Chris Dittmar was there all the time with us, intimidating as ever but a great player and training incredibly hard. He was from Adelaide, where the world open was being held, and he obviously wanted to do well in his home town. I remember playing practice matches with him where immediately afterwards he would take on somebody else. He would often spend 40 minutes practising on his own as well – and all this after a gruelling training session in the morning. During the practice matches, most of the top players like the Martins and Rodney Eyles were more concerned about working on their game than they were with winning, but not Dittmar. Even when there was nothing at stake, he was determined to give us a good pasting.

I learnt a tremendous amount during those two weeks, which is just as well because I was about to face the biggest challenge of my career so far. Lying in wait at the world open was a very special player who was more formidable than everyone at the institute put together.

# 4.

## BEATING KING KHAN

Forget the mighty Liverpool FC and their domination of football in the early '80s; never mind Ian Botham and his ability to win test matches on his own; don't worry either about Seve Ballesteros playing impossible golf shots or Steve Davis potting everyone off the snooker table at around the same time. All of these great sportsmen were, of course, way ahead of their challengers. But for all their undeniable brilliance, none of them dominated their chosen field as much as Jahingir Khan dominated the world of squash. Not since the days of Muhammad Ali has one man reigned so supreme as a champion among champions.

As part of the year 2000 celebrations, Jahingir was voted Pakistan's Sportsman of the Millennium. That's an impressive honour by any standards, but particularly so in a cricket-mad country that has produced such world-class names as Imran Khan, Wasim Akram and Wakir Younis. All of those great stars, together with top squash players from around the world, gathered in Pakistan to pay tribute to Jahingir at the award ceremony. It was yet another pinnacle in a career that had begun more than 20 years earlier, when in 1979 he was sent by Pakistan International Airlines, a major sponsor of sport in Pakistan, to compete in the world championships in Australia. Nothing much was expected of him and he was there mainly to get some experience. He got plenty of experience all right – he won the tournament. He was just 15 at the time, the youngest champion ever. The world of squash was made to sit up and take notice of the name Jahingir Khan.

When he won, Jahinger was as surprised as anyone but the victory gave him a great deal of self-belief. He set about demolishing top professionals in the same way he had cut down the top amateurs. At times, he seemed like a man possessed. His determination and dedication may have owed something to the tragic death of his brother Torsam. Torsam was a very good player himself at that time, but he was coming to the end of his career. His main ambition was to coach and guide Jahingir to the world number one spot. He set out to play one last tournament in Australia before retiring to concentrate on coaching. Tragically, he died on court. He and Torsam had been very close and Jahingir was unable to play or think of anything but his brother for several months. Eventually, he emerged from his mourning more determined than ever to become world number one, not only for himself but also for his brother, who had shown such faith in him.

In the space of just two years, he was to become the best player in the world. After winning the world amateur title, he spent a summer in England training with Jonah Barrington. They played each other three times a week in practice matches. At the start of the summer, Jonah could cope with him quite comfortably. But he described afterwards how he could see Jahingir getting better and better as the weeks went by. He started playing with the kind of pace and power that left Jonah struggling. By the end of the summer, Jonah could just about hold on to him but had to push himself to the limits to do it. He witnessed at first hand an incredible rate of improvement. Jonah said he knew straight away that Jahinger would not only be world champion, he would be something very special for a long time.

Jahingir left England that summer a much stronger player, ready to take on anyone, and quickly established himself as a major force in the game. Then, in 1981, he played another squash legend – Geoff Hunt. He lost 3–1 in a gruelling game that lasted nearly two and a half hours. It was a major landmark in the history of squash, for it was to be another 800 games and over five and a half years before Jahingir lost again. That's a record no one has come close to matching before or since. He was unstoppable. World-class players like Ross Norman and Chris Dittmar have described how they and fellow professionals would meet and discuss possible ways to beat him. They had lots of ideas – but none of them worked.

There was quite a contrast between Jahingir the man and Jahingir the player. Off court, he was polite and softly spoken, self-effacing and quiet to the point of shyness. He didn't mix very much with the other players and tended to content himself with the company of the large entourage that followed him around. On court, however, he turned into a formidable athlete who was totally ruthless in destroying opponents. His fitness level seemed superhuman and he would fight every point as if to the death. There was certainly the air of the warrior about him and he showed his opponents no mercy. I witnessed his ruthlessness first-hand at the age of nine, when I saw him for the first time. He was playing Maxim Ahmed in the final of a world professional association tournament. Jahingir's performance was breathtaking. He won 9–0, 9–0, 9–0. Poor Ahmed was powerless to do anything about it. It was like watching a lamb being taken for slaughter.

No one can maintain a machine-like consistency forever, of course, and defeat had to come eventually. The New Zealander Ross Norman was the man to inflict the damage. Norman was a fantastic battler. He became the world number two and spent much of his career losing to Jahingir in the finals of all the major events around the world. However, no matter how much he was outclassed, he always gave 100 per cent. His philosophy was that if he could keep playing at the top of his game then one day Jahingir would have an off-day and he would beat him. For years, it seemed a forlorn hope but then the impossible happened. Norman got his reward when he ended Jahingir's five-and-a-half-year run with a victory in the final of the World Open in 1986. It was such a shock that it made headline news all over the world. I heard it on the BBC nine o'clock television news which doesn't normally mention minority sports like squash.

There was no doubting Jahingir's dominance at this time, but it must also be remembered that the overall standard of the game at top level wasn't as high as it had been a few years earlier or was about to become a few years later. By the early '80s stars like Barrington and Hunt had retired, leaving a vacuum that only Jahingir seemed capable of filling. There was a gap of three or four years before the next set of world class performers arrived on the scene in the shape of Ross Norman, and then Rod Martin and Chris Dittmar. They were a younger breed who hadn't played him when he was at his peak very often, and so hadn't been bludgeoned into a belief that he couldn't be beaten. In the intervening period Jahingir was so far ahead of everyone else that many people were almost beaten before they even went on court. It meant they didn't push him as far as they could because they thought they had no chance of winning.

I was impressed at the time by Jahingir's unbeaten run, but after turning professional I came to appreciate it even more. You really need to feel 100 per cent to perform at your best on a consistent basis, yet there are so many days when you don't feel particularly well. You might have a little injury or be recovering from some minor illness, or whatever. That must have happened to Jahingir several times over that five-year period yet he kept on winning, most of the time without even dropping a game.

Jahingir took his defeat by Norman with good grace, acknowledging that players can't always be the same day in, day out. He was also aware that many people had stopped coming to tournaments to see him win. They were coming to see him lose, as is inevitable when a champion moves so far ahead of the field. It was a great victory for Norman and although Jahingir continued to win far more often than he lost, his air of invincibility was gone. Soon Rod Martin and Chris Dittmar were ready to battle with him. Ironically, their emergence probably made Jahingir an even better player than he was before. They were good enough to test him and so helped him to improve. They weren't as in awe of him as players had been a few years earlier, and they did manage to beat him occasionally. They couldn't stop him collecting a record ten consecutive British Open titles, however, as well as winning every other major tournament over and over again.

There's no doubt that Jahingir took the game to a new level. He was my boyhood hero. I remember going to watch the British Open championships with my dad and being amazed that Jahingir was there in real life, only a few yards away from me. He was the most famous squash player since Jonah Barrington. I was in awe of him when I was younger, but having turned professional I had to look at him differently. He was the man I most wanted to beat and then emulate. I never thought I would be one of the last people to defeat him before he retired from the game.

I first met Jahinger in Australia in the last 16 of the World Open in 1991. As soon as the draw was made, some people started commiserating with me for my misfortune in drawing Jahingir. Such was his stature that they thought I was unlucky to have to meet him so early in the tournament. I didn't see it that way at all. I was really excited at the prospect of playing him, and couldn't wait to get on court. It was important to me to test myself against the best. I always felt that way if I was drawn against a top player. It would annoy other people because they would see it as certain defeat, but I didn't care about that. I knew I would probably lose but still looked forward to the game. I regarded it as an opportunity to learn from a better player and so improve my game. It was a bit purist, perhaps, but that's how I saw it.

I was doing well at the time: I was the England number one and ranked 15 in the world. I had enjoyed a meteoric rise up the rankings during the previous 18 months, despite falling behind my friend and rival Simon Parke for a while. I had been ahead of Simon for most of our early years, but he beat me to the England number one spot even though he was younger than me, only 19 at the time. Having achieved so much so young he might have been expected to zoom forward to greater things, but he didn't, not immediately anyway. Instead, he seemed to lose focus. By his own admission, he rested on his laurels for a while. He started going out a lot more and developed other interests.

Looking back, this seems to me a perfectly natural and healthy thing to do, but for some reason I didn't follow the same path. I did go out and socialise, of course, but not as much as Simon and certainly not as much as most other people of the same age. I remained more focused on squash. You have to be determined to succeed, and at that time I was probably more determined than most. There were several reasons for this. I always loved playing and took a lot of satisfaction in finding ways to improve. Getting better was almost more important than winning. Part of me would have preferred to play well and lose than to play badly and win. Maybe that was a purist approach, but I had been that way since childhood. I'm not sure where it came from, but it had spurred me on throughout my career. It meant I was always prepared to work that bit harder and apply myself that little bit more than others.

I was also aware even then that I wasn't the most talented player on the circuit. I probably didn't have as much skill as Simon, and certainly didn't have as much as 'flair players' like Brett Martin. I wasn't a great athlete in terms of speed or grace or racket skills. My greatest asset was my mental strength. I could apply myself and keep going through the pain barrier and beyond when others might give in. I knew that success for me could only come through hard work and supreme physical fitness. I didn't have the same margin for error that others might have, so I had to be more dedicated.

It may be that part of me was also motivated by the need to answer those people who had criticised my two-handed style. I had become tired of people telling me it would never work at the top level. It was bad enough as a junior, but it continued even when I was a senior. I remember playing Simon at a tournament in Harrogate when I was about 18. One of the top England players at the time, Ian Robinson, had a word with me afterwards, urging me to change. He said it might work at junior level but that the top professionals would find it too easy to exploit. I found that irritating, as I always did, and I suppose the continual criticism became yet another motivating force for me. Press cuttings of my early career were often dominated by headlines such as 'Marshall defies his critics' every time I won a match against a top player.

I was also naturally ambitious, of course, and wanted to get to the top. As I got to the end of my teens, I felt pressure to do well and improve. Part of it was down to drawing comparisons between myself and other players. I was impressed by people like Del Harris, who had become England number one at the age of 18 and remained there for two or three years. He got into the world top ten soon afterwards. I realised that my eighteenth birthday had come and gone and I hadn't achieved nearly as much. It was worse when I looked at the likes of Jahingir and Jansher Khan, who had become world champions while still in their teens. I felt I should be achieving more and I was driven to work harder. Of course, I never compared myself to players who weren't doing as well as I was; only those who were doing better.

It's likely that I had developed a greater sense of urgency because of the bout of glandular fever, which gave me a sense that I had fallen behind and needed to make up for lost time. I compensated by working even harder. In retrospect, it's easy to see that I probably put too much pressure on myself. I tried to do too much too soon. It would have been hard to sustain if I had been in perfect health, but looking back I suspect that I wasn't in perfect health at all. It's impossible to draw definite conclusions even now, but I feel there was something simmering away beneath the surface. There were the bouts of tonsillitis that had returned with monotonous regularity each year throughout my childhood, the glandular fever and then the occasional but regular periods when I would feel under the weather without being able to put my finger on exactly what was wrong. There were also the times when I got colds and flu. These minor illnesses afflict everyone at times, of course, but I seemed more prone to them than most. This was even more surprising when you consider that I was young and fit and worked hard to keep myself in good condition. The illnesses could be very frustrating, like the time I had to pull out of the US Open. I would always be counting the days until I could get back to work. Perhaps I was coming back too soon at times.

With the benefit of hindsight, I can see that there was a disaster waiting to happen. At the time, however, I was blissfully unaware that I might be creating problems for myself. Each month brought an exciting new adventure to occupy my mind; it could be a new tournament, or a visit to an exotic country I had never been to before. Best of all was the thrill of pitting my wits against a big-name player. And, of course, they didn't come any bigger than Jahingir Khan. It would have been wonderful merely to play him back home in Nottingham in a practice match with nobody watching; to meet him in the World Open in a glamorous venue thousands of miles from home was like heaven to me. I couldn't wait for match day to arrive.

Surprisingly, I wasn't at all daunted at the prospect of playing him. I almost developed a blind belief that I could beat him. Perhaps he's not that good, I told myself. It wasn't confidence as much as a sense that anything could happen. Fellow professionals tried to bring me back down to earth. I had played most of the top players by then, but they all warned me that playing Jahingir would be a totally new experience. It was something that couldn't be described, they said. You simply had to play him to understand it.

It only took a few moments on court with him to realise what they meant. He played to a standard I had never encountered before. It was strange, because it could be said that I should have known exactly what to expect. I had studied his game, and in many ways I had modelled myself on him. I wanted to play in a similar way. I knew his strengths inside out, yet, no matter how much I knew about him, it still came as a surprise to be on court with him and experience it for real. I couldn't prevent myself being totally obliterated. I lost in about 40 minutes without getting anywhere near him. Whatever I did, he had an answer. He gave me no time to think, react or do anything. Wherever I placed the ball, he was there. It was like trying to get past a brick wall. It reminded me of the time when I was about 12, playing men for the first time, struggling to cope with their pace and power. It was very frustrating. I came off court feeling inadequate and totally demoralised. I kept telling myself: 'This is supposed to be your profession, and you've been made to look like a beginner.' I was 20 at the time and it made me realise that although I was heading towards the world top ten, there was still a huge gap between me and Jahingir.

Those thoughts didn't last for long, however. I knew I had to keep the defeat in perspective and put it down to experience. I wasn't the only player to take a thumping from him. There was a huge gap between Jahingir and all the world's leading players at that time. I reminded myself that I had only been on the professional circuit for a few years and he was the greatest player the game had ever produced. I hadn't been expected to do well against him. On the positive side, I knew I had learnt a great deal from the match. In squash, as in most sports, you improve by playing better players. In unequal matches, the weaker player who loses is likely to learn far more from the experience than the stronger player who wins. I knew I could advance an enormous amount just from that one match against Jahingir, agonising though it was.

It wasn't hard to analyse Jahingir's game. Although he was quite small, he was solid and compact. He was surprisingly strong and powerful, both physically and mentally. Like so many of the great champions, his game was based on shots played hard and accurate into the back corners. The biggest difference I noticed in playing him, however, was the faster pace of the game. That's probably the main thing you notice when you step up in standard in all sports. The ball is taken much earlier. He saw things very quickly, and would move on to the ball and volley it; he didn't like to let shots go past him and then play them off the back wall. This meant he seemed to play every shot a fraction of a second earlier than other players did, and so you had less time to react. I quickly realised that with him the little errors that other players weren't quick enough to exploit were immediately seized upon and exploited. It gave me a lot to think about. As at all levels, it's only by competing against better players that you see where your game breaks down, whether technically or physically. Jahingir made me appreciate, as if for the first time, the value of the simple basics played quickly and accurately. I went away determined to improve.

First, though, I wanted to watch the rest of the tournament and take the rare opportunity to spend a few days relaxing with my parents. They had travelled to Australia in a somewhat unusual manner. My dad had sold the club at Kegworth a few years earlier and retired, which gave him time to concentrate on his new sporting passion, sailing. He'd taken it up late in life but in his usual way he threw himself into it and learned very quickly. Every summer when I was a child we would go sailing for most of the summer holidays. Since Dad didn't have much experience, we started off sailing to places like France. Soon after, he graduated to the Greek islands and all around the Mediterranean. Then, with a few more years' experience behind him after retiring, he was ready for a bigger challenge. He and Mum decided to sail around the world. It meant I didn't get to see them all that often, and they weren't able to follow my squash career as closely as before. Fortunately, they were able to catch up with me as I prepared to play that World Open match against Jahingir. As chance would have it, they were passing Adelaide at that time and called in to see me.

It was good to have them in my corner again, just like the old days when I was a junior. It gave me a boost to see them and I couldn't help but admire their courage in taking on such a daunting task. They had sold the house and now lived permanently on the boat. I stayed in Adelaide with them for a few days and managed to follow the rest of the tournament. To my surprise, Jahingir didn't go on to win it. Neither did that other Pakistani legend, Jansher Khan. They both lost to the eventual winner, Rod Martin. That was a fantastic achievement on his part. Until then no one had beaten both Khans in the same tournament. Martin also threw in a fantastic win over Chris Dittmar as well. The squash he played that week was probably the best I have ever seen. From watching Martin and playing Jahingir, I probably got enough inspiration that week to last a lifetime.

I spent a few more days with my parents and then we parted to go our separate ways. Their voyage was to take them across the Great Australian Bight and its shark infested waters, then 4,000 miles across the Indian Ocean to South Africa. After taking in stops at places like Perth along the way, they reckoned it would take them the best part of a year. That meant they should be arriving along the African coast by the following September. By a happy coincidence, the 1992 World Open was being held in Johannesburg at that time and they said they'd stop by to see me again.

Despite developing sea legs, Dad still liked his squash and missed watching the tournaments.

I headed back to Europe to compete in an invitation tournament. When I got there, I started to feel unwell. I thought perhaps I was coming down with flu again but thankfully it didn't turn out to be that bad. Nevertheless, I was tired and felt weaker and more listless than usual. It didn't stop me playing and I managed to get to the final, although it all seemed much more of an effort than usual. I eventually lost to Ross Norman. He was a great player, so it was no real surprise, but I still felt disappointed. I felt that I hadn't been able to give it my best shot because of the way I was feeling.

There was no point in dwelling on it too long. I wanted to get back to England for a relaxing Christmas break. After that, it would be time to prepare for the British National Championships in January. The tournament had seemed a bit jinxed for me in previous years. I was disqualified in 1988 for arriving late for a match after getting stuck in a traffic jam. In 1991, I had to withdraw after suffering from food poisoning. I thought it was about time I got a decent break, but I returned home to find there was yet more jinx potential in the making. I had worked my way up the rankings and was now the British number one. Consequently, I was put down as the top seed. Obviously that would normally be considered a good thing, but the championships had proved something of a graveyard for the favourites – the previous three tournaments had all been won by outsiders!

The toughest game of the tournament was likely to be against Simon Parke who I was due to play in the semi-final, assuming all went to plan for both of us. We both had relatively easy victories in the first round. I beat Rick Weatherall in straight sets. Simon had a similarly straightforward victory over an up-and-coming young lad from Scotland called Peter Nicol. What we'd all give for an easy straight sets victory over him now! Thankfully, the jinx didn't kick in for me that year. I met Simon in the semis as expected and managed to win 3–0. The score didn't really do justice to Simon. It was a momentous battle, and it took me more than 80 minutes to win through. I played some of the best squash of my career so far. The experience against Jahingir had definitely strengthened my game.

In the final, I came up against Brian Beeson. He had won the tournament in 1986, but like every champion since Jonny Leslie, who won the first British Closed in 1974, he had failed to defend it successfully. There was definitely something about that tournament that didn't like top seeds! I lost the first game but then came back strongly to win the next three. The final two games were both 9–0 and demonstrated that my game had moved up several notches since playing Jahingir. Beeson was very complimentary afterwards, saying: 'Marshall is amazing. Just getting the service from him is like striking gold.'

I was delighted with the victory. It was the third and most satisfying landmark of my early career: the first was breaking into the main tournaments and playing top stars like Dittmar and Robertson; the second was the Canadian Open when I got past the early rounds for the first time and beat some of the top seeds. Those performances made people notice me and comment that I had the potential to do well. I wanted more than that, however. I wanted to make that potential a reality. Becoming British National Champion went a long way towards achieving that ambition.

The victory confirmed my position as the British number one. A few people had questioned whether I should have been the top seed, and winning the tournament was the best way of demonstrating that I was there on merit. The £3,000 prize money was also very welcome. It was a good week's work. I couldn't dwell on it too long, however, and had to leave my celebration party early that night to make sure I would be in good shape for a Yorkshire league match the following night. British champion or not, I still had to continue with the bread and butter work.

On a more glamorous note, I had big tournaments coming up in Germany, Spain and France. I would be going there with renewed confidence, looking to improve my world ranking. There was also the possibility of earning a lot more money. The game was richer than it had ever been before. The British Open, to be held in April, had a prize fund of over £100,000. Worldwide, the total prize money available on the circuit was set to exceed £1 million for the first time. The game was very strong and the timing was perfect for young English players like me and Simon Parke who were starting to emerge at the top level.

---

The year 1991 was a good one for me and by the autumn, I had broken into the world top ten. It was another huge landmark. I'm not sure if I realised it at the time, but those rankings were significant for reasons that had nothing to do with me: for the first time in nearly ten years, Jahingir Khan fell from the number one spot. His place was taken by Jansher Khan. Chris Dittmar was ranked second with Rod Martin third. Chris Robertson was fourth. Jahingir could only manage fifth place. It was the end of an era, for the great man would never again regain the number one position. It was the beginning of the age of Jansher Khan. The new rankings were confirmation that while my career had soared since playing Jahingir only six months earlier, his by contrast was starting to show signs of cracks. He was troubled by a niggling back injury that was taking a long time to clear up. He'd had to withdraw from that year's British Open because of it. It meant he missed the chance to notch up his eleventh consecutive title.

There was also a feeling among some of the top players that Jahingir wasn't quite as hungry as he used to be. He was only really motivated for the top two or three tournaments — hardly surprising after all he had achieved. Whether he had lost some of his appetite or it was due to his back injury, there was no doubt that he had lost some of his edge and wasn't quite as formidable as he had been at his peak. Jahinger was still winning most of his matches, but the games were getting closer. There were times when he was in and out of form and sometimes he would arrive at tournaments looking a bit overweight. Some people said they also noticed a change in his attitude. He had always been fair on court, didn't dispute anything and just got on with the game. I certainly had no problem with him when I'd played him the previous year. However, other players felt that as he got older he had to use a little gamesmanship now and then to get through. There was always a lot of friction when he came up against the other outstanding player of that era, Rod Martin. Those were often niggly matches, with Martin accusing Jahingir of not getting out of the way fast enough and standing on his shots. It got to a point where they hardly spoke to each other.

Jahingir's back injury kept him out of the game for about six months over the summer of 1992. However, he was back on the circuit and apparently fully fit by the time of World Open in September. It was a very special occasion, because it was to be held in South Africa: for nearly 20 years, the country's apartheid laws had led to sanctions, giving it an outcast status. An international boycott prevented South Africa taking part in international sports tournaments; no major events were held there. However, by the early '90s all that was changing. Nelson Mandela had been released from prison and was about to become president. South Africa was welcomed back into the international fold. The World Open squash tournament was one of the first international events to be held there since the lifting of the boycott.

This was a great boost for South Africa and a wonderful opportunity for young players like me to visit the country for the first time. I went out two weeks before the tournament with the England squad to get used to the climate, particularly the high altitude. The place was a little scary at first; there was still a great deal of unrest following the political changes. A couple of tournament officials were beaten up one night and we were advised not to go out. We quickly got used to it, though, and I still remember it as one of the most beautiful places I've ever visited. We stayed with a family who made us very welcome and for those two warm-up weeks, we enjoyed a very relaxed lifestyle.

Then came the serious business of the tournament. It was a case of history repeating itself. I was drawn to play Jahingir again in the last 16. And, just as my parents had turned up just in time to watch the match a year earlier in Adelaide, so they arrived right on cue to see the game in Johannesburg. It was a serious case of déjà vu, but this time I was determined that the result would be different. I was confident that this time I might beat Jahingir. I had improved enormously in the 12 months since our last match. I was more experienced, my matchplay was better and, of course, I was a year older. That may not seem significant, but a year makes a huge difference at that age. I was fitter and much stronger. By contrast, Jahingir seemed to be going in the opposite direction. He may have only been 28 but he had been on the circuit for 12 gruelling years.

Jahinger was the kind of player who believed in total fitness and he had pushed his body to its limits all his life. And as he went all the way to the final in nearly every tournament, he rarely had much time to rest before flying out to yet another country to do it all over again. His spectacular success meant that most of his career had been spent in the media spotlight. Squash is enormous in Pakistan and he was treated like a superstar, recognised and fêted wherever he went. It sounds glamorous, but it can also be wearying. That kind of lifestyle is bound to take its toll on anyone. I wondered about his ability to keep pushing himself through yet more hurdles to win titles he'd already won several times before.

Jahingir looked all right as he arrived in Johannesburg. His coach boasted that the great man was fitter and stronger than he had ever been. I wasn't convinced. His six months out left him very little time to prepare properly and get his body in peak condition. He hadn't had the chance to play many games before the tournament, so I felt sure he wouldn't be fully match fit. I watched him in his first-round match against the German number one, Hansi Weins. Weins was in the world top 20 and a very useful player. Jahingir won 3–0 but I felt he looked a bit rusty; I spoke to Weins afterwards, and he agreed. He thought I had a good chance of winning.

I thought my best chance would be to try to expose Jahinger's lack of fitness. The fact that we were playing at an altitude where the air was thinner would make it even more physically demanding. My game plan was therefore quite straightforward. I knew I had to keep the rallies going, and keep him moving on court for as long as possible. This would make him work so that he would tire. It was vital to keep him away from the front of the court where he was lethal with tight drop shots. These were hard enough to get to at the best of times, but as he got older and slower, he didn't get out of the way as quickly as he used to do. This meant you sometimes had to go round him to get to the ball, making it even more difficult to retrieve his shot. That was one of the things Rod Martin always complained about. However, I was reasonably confident of doing well – and the longer the game went on the more my chances would increase, as I was physically stronger.

It was ironic that, although I was the up-and-coming newcomer, it was Jahingir who was more of an unknown quantity at that time. Because of his injuries, no one quite knew what to expect. There were question marks over his mental strength as well. He had retired from a few matches when they had become close and physically demanding. There was a lot of interest in how he would perform and most of the top players came to watch the match.

It worked out very well for me. For most of the first hour of the game Jahingir played with his usual skill and pace, but he wasn't dominating me the way he had the year before. He had lost a bit of speed around the court and wasn't getting out of the corners fast enough. I felt he was getting in my way, which I found very irritating. It was strange in a way. A few years before, as a squash fan, I had been in awe of him. It was amazing to think that I now saw him as just another person I happened to be competing against. He was even annoying me!

Jahinger took the first two games, but they were very close: 15–12 and 15–13. I could sense that he was tiring towards the end of the second game and felt that if I could manage to stay with him then I would still have a chance. Phil Whitlock, who had been in the world top ten, came down from the stands to give me some advice. He urged me keep the ball away from Jahingir for as long as possible. He was still devastating with the racket, and was able to hit outright winners off any loose cross-court shots. He was quite big at this point and it was difficult to get round him to hit the ball. Whitlock told me to hit every shot straight down the walls for the first ten minutes no matter what. It was probably the best single piece of advice anyone ever gave me. I did exactly what Whitlock said and for the next two games I played some of the best squash of my life. It had an immediate effect. I could see Jahingir having to work harder and he was tiring. He wasn't nearly as strong in that third game and I took it relatively easily, 15–2.

I won the next game 15–7 and felt that Jahingir was really struggling with the pace. He was starting to hold his back at times as if it was troubling him again. At 6–9 down, he called for a let but the referee refused to grant it. That really annoyed him and, unusually for him, he questioned the decision, even going off the court and inviting the referee to play in his place. He seemed to lose heart after that and lost the remaining points very easily. Some people commented afterwards that I seemed to grow tense as the prospect of victory became more of a reality. I don't know about that, but it's not every day you get the chance to secure victory against the greatest player in the world! There was one awkward moment when I felt Jahingir wasn't getting out of the way quickly enough and accused him of blocking me. I was so annoyed I threw my racket down in fury and was given a code of conduct warning. Perhaps nerves were getting a bit fraught on both sides.

I was looking forward to the fifth game and felt sure I would win when

Jahingir stunned me and everyone else by conceding the match. He simply walked back on court after the break, shook hands with me and then walked away to his dressing-room. He said his back injury had flared up again and he couldn't continue. I was disappointed because I felt I had been denied a proper victory. It would have been great to have gone all the way and got the final point against him, but it wasn't to be. I'm still going to claim it as a real victory, however, as I had done all I could and got my tactics right. There's no doubt that he had gone downhill a little, but then I had improved enormously – perhaps we met somewhere in the middle.

The crowd were warm in their applause though perhaps a little sad to see the match end that way. Chris Dittmar was one of the first people to congratulate me. He had played Jahingir several times and knew how tough he was. Most of the other players who were watching were also pleased that I had won. Many were sceptical, however, about Jahingir's withdrawal due to injury. They felt he could have played on but stopped because he knew he was going to be beaten. Simon Parke was there and said the great man had gone down a little in the estimation of his fellow professionals. I don't know whether Jahingir could have carried on, and I suppose I never will. Whatever the case, beating him that day remains one of the highlights of my career. It was certainly my greatest achievement up to that point, even better than becoming British Champion.

After the euphoria of beating Jahingir, I was quickly brought down to earth when I lost in the quarter-final against Austin Adaragga. It was disappointing after beating Jahinger, but that's the way the game goes sometimes. I had to console myself with the fact that at least I had become one of the few players in the world to beat Jahingir. He continued to struggle with his fitness for the following few months. He played a few more tournaments the following year but his injuries recurred and he finally retired. Everyone was very sorry to see him go because he had been a wonderful player and a great boost for the game. He had emerged just as Jonah Barrington was starting to fade, at a time when squash needed another great character to capture the public imagination. Jahingir filled that role perfectly and helped fuel the squash boom that swept the world in the '80s. Like Jonah, he brought the game to a new level by setting a standard that other players had to strive to meet.

After retiring from the game, he returned to Pakistan where he still lives with his wife and daughter. In traditional Pakistani style, they're part of an extended family consisting of his parents, together with his brother and his wife and children. His father Roshan, who won the British Open in 1957, is at the head of the household. In 1999, Jahingir was appointed the vice president of the World Squash Federation.

I enjoyed my two matches against him and would have liked to play him many more times but, sadly, it wasn't to be. Soon, however, I came up against another mighty Pakistani, Jansher Khan – no relation to Jahingir, but equally formidable in his own way. For the next three years, we were to slug it out across five continents, producing some of the best matches of that period. My determination to beat Jansher inspired me to produce the best squash of my career. I fear it also helped to bring about my downfall.

# 5.

## THE EASTERN MASTER

There are many ways an up-and-coming teenager might react after being demolished by the greatest player his sport has ever seen. He might feel crushed and decide he never wanted to play again. Someone else would probably see it as a learning experience and vow to keep working so he could do better in a few years time. The young Jansher Khan, however, took a different approach. When he was 17, he lost quite easily against Jahingir. Instead of coming out with the usual niceties about what a great honour it was to play him and how much he had learnt from the experience, he made a startling prediction. He promised he would beat Jahingir within six months and then overtake him as the world's best player.

Some people were outraged at such impudence; others merely amused at such youthful delusion. No one believed him. Jansher, however, was as good as his word. Shortly afterwards he beat Jahingir 3–0 in the final of the Hong Kong Open. He then went on to beat him consistently and replaced him as the world number one, exactly as he said he would. Everyone was astonished. Only two players had beaten Jahingir at that time, Ross Norman and Rodney Martin. And they had only managed it once each. No one had beaten him consistently, yet here was this teenager running up a string of victories. Jansher beat Jahingir nine times in their first eleven meetings. Their games were often long, and frustrating for Jahingir. Sometimes he would go 2–0 up and might even have match ball. But Jansher would come back at him and go on to win.

Unfortunately for Jansher, his success didn't win him many friends back home in Pakistan; at least, not in those early days. He was seen as the brash young upstart who was taking the crown of the much loved Jahingir. It was almost considered improper and the fans didn't like it. He had to suffer the indignity of being booed after beating Jahingir in the final of the Pakistan Open. There were many reasons for this. The final was played in Karachi, which was home territory for Jahingir. Jansher was from Peshawar and seen as a bit of an outsider. Another factor was Jansher's personality; or rather, the way his personality was perceived by others. Jahingir had been considered the perfect professional and the ultimate sportsman. He was shy, but diplomatic and always said the right things. Jansher, by contrast, was more outspoken and had a tendency to make controversial statements. The prediction that he would beat Jahingir was considered arrogant and disrespectful to a great champion. He made matters worse after the Pakistan Open final by saying he now had the measure of Jahingir and would continue to beat him. The fact that it turned out to be true only added to some people's irritation.

Jansher could also get on the wrong side of sponsors and tournament organisers. There was one story of how he had supposedly upset people at the celebration banquet after the World Championships in Kuala Lumpur in 1989. As world champion, Jansher was the guest of honour, seated next to the chairman of the company sponsoring the tournament. Unfortunately he was late for the meal, keeping the distinguished guests waiting. When he did finally turn up he wasn't considered properly dressed for a formal dinner and had also brought some of his entourage with him. They hadn't been invited and were apparently noisy and unwelcome. The organisers were so angry they delayed paying him his prize money and considered disciplinary action.

There were also times when he played league matches for clubs but gave the impression that he was not trying as hard as he might, although on most occasions he did play well. That could be disappointing for fans who had made a special effort to see him. To be fair, though, it's hard for any player to be at his best all the time. Everyone needs to plan their programme so that they peak in the big tournaments. That doesn't always coincide with being on top form in exhibition games or club matches. The problem was probably highlighted by the fact that he was the world champion and world number one: people expected him to be devastating all the time. If other players did badly, no one thought anything of it, but when Jansher slipped below his usual high standard it received much more attention.

Throughout his career, he often made seemingly dismissive statements about other players. On one occasion, he beat Zarak Jahan Khan and afterwards suggested that he wasn't a very good player and Jansher could beat him anytime, anywhere. When he was only 17, he was drawn to play Chris Dittmar in the British Open. Dittmar was one of the best players in the world at the time, yet Jansher made out he had never heard of him. He said something like: 'I'm playing some redheaded Australian guy, but I don't know who he is.' This didn't go down well with people and it certainly meant that he and Dittmar weren't going to get on well. The two of them went on to have a long rivalry and the animosity between them remained throughout their careers. It was made worse because Dittmar became president of the Professional Squash Association. Part of his job was to promote the game and keep sponsors happy, and he didn't think Jansher was good for the game because he didn't portray a good image.

Jansher's comments about other players may have come across as arrogant, but I believe they were nearly all tongue in cheek. He had a lively sense of humour which people sometimes failed to recognise, perhaps because he kept apart from other players at tournaments which made it hard to get to know him. He just liked to get the job done and stay within his own entourage. He didn't give much away in press interviews either, so it was hard to find out what he really thought about things.

I played Jansher 15 times and never had any trouble with him. He always treated me with respect although he sometimes engaged in a bit of banter after the match. I remember him telling me once that he would thrash me easily in the next big tournament we played. His tone was similar to the one he had adopted when making remarks about Dittmar or Khan. I took him to be joking. Maybe he was trying to wind me up, but I don't think he meant any harm and I certainly didn't take it that way. I think he was the same throughout his career. You might not think his sense of humour was particularly funny, but I'm sure there was no malice or genuine disrespect in it.

On another occasion, I remember talking to him about my two-handed style. He first saw me play at a tournament in Norfolk when I was 18, in which he was supporting my opponent that day, Zarak Jahan Khan. Jansher told me he had heard that I played two-handed but didn't believe it was possible, and that when he saw me knocking up before the game he almost started laughing because it looked so strange. He thought I was going to get hammered, but soon changed his mind once the game got underway. Zarak was a top player but I took a 2–1 lead before he came back to take the match. I ran him very close considering I was only 18. Jansher stopped laughing after that because he realised I could play. Again, I suppose I could have taken offence at Jansher's apparently dismissive attitude towards my technique, but I don't think he meant any harm.

It's a great pity that Jansher came across badly to some people, particularly in his own country, because it meant he didn't get the recognition he deserved. While Jahingir was being honoured as Pakistan's sportsman of the century, Jansher was left out in the cold. He didn't even come into the reckoning, which is ridiculous, really; there was very little between the two players and their achievements.

I first saw Jansher when he played in the British Open in 1987. He was only 17 and it was his first appearance in the competition. He amazed everyone by getting to the final. In his trail he left some of the greatest players of the day: Rodney Eyles, Zarak Jahan Khan, Gawain Briers, Ross Norman (the reigning world champion at that time), and 'that redheaded Australian', Chris Dittmar. He played Jahingir in the final and I remembered being fascinated by the contrast in their styles. Jahingir played his usual game, based on all-out blitzkrieg attack.

Jansher could not have been more different. He opposed Jahingir's hard, fast pace by slowing the game down completely. He had a game that no one had used for a long time, using lots of lobs to the back of the court and giving the opponent very little opportunity to attack from the front. The most amazing thing about him, however, was the way he covered the court so easily. For much of the time, he seemed to be walking about. Even Jahingir sometimes looked hurried, as though he was finding it difficult to get to the ball. For Jansher, it always seemed to be a gentle stroll. I don't know how he did it. Perhaps it was incredible anticipation or maybe he just had very quick feet. Whatever it was, nothing seemed to ruffle him. I have never seen anyone with such good movement and I doubt if I ever will again.

Despite Jansher's obvious brilliance, he was still only 17 and it was his first British Open. Jahingir won 3–0. Shortly afterwards, Jansher made his notorious prediction. I think everyone realised during that tournament that a major new force had arrived. The next few years were to turn into something of a golden age for squash. Not only did we have the mighty Khans, but a trio of top flight Australians: Rodney Martin, Chris Dittmar and Chris Robertson. Such coincidences occur perhaps only once in a generation in any given sport. It happened in tennis with players like Jimmy Connors, Bjorn Borg and John McEnroe. Their epic battles evoke stirring memories even now, and such is their appeal that they can still pull big crowds when they play veterans' matches. Athletics had a golden period with the rivalry between Sebastian Coe, Steve Ovett and Steve Cram. The competition between those three attracted the attention of people who wouldn't normally show any interest in middle distance running.

I have to admit to feeling slightly sorry for Martin, Dittmar and Robertson. They were three fantastic players who would have dominated the game at any other time. As it turned out, they had to spend most of their careers fighting each other for second place behind their rivals from Pakistan. Can you imagine the frustration they must have felt? They had spent years losing to Jahingir and no doubt looking forward to the moment when he would retire. Then, just as it seemed he might be showing signs of easing up, another equally formidable star emerged. It was tough on them, but it was great for squash because it led to some fantastic matches.

By the time I was 19, I was looking forward to taking part in some great matches myself. I got my first chance against Jansher in the second round of the Leekes Welsh Classic in Cardiff in 1991. This was before my first game with Jahingir and was therefore played at a standard that I had never encountered before. I had no fears. I never did when I came up against the top players, because that was where I wanted to be. It was totally different from playing Jahingir for the first time, or even the other top players like Robertson and Dittmar. Jansher didn't put you under any great pressure in the way they did. He didn't hit the ball hard or take it particularly early. You always felt as though you were in the rally and might get him out of position at any moment and hit a winner. Somehow, though, you hardly ever managed to do that. There was nothing spectacular about him but whatever you did, he seemed to have an answer for it. I quickly realised that hitting a winner against him was a major achievement. He seemed to pick everything up. It was very frustrating because in every rally he seemed to be able to play just one more shot than you could. It was amazing really. Where Jahingir was an out-and-out aggressive street fighter who would take the game to anyone, Jansher was more of a defensive counter puncher. He would let you take the initiative and then react.

As everyone expected at that time, I was beaten 3–0 but took comfort in the fact that I had made one of the greatest players of all time fight all the way. It took Jansher 72 minutes to subdue me. And with the scores at 15–13, 15–10 and 15–12, it was hardly a walkover. In the typically British style of supporting the underdog, the press reported the game as if I had won. *The Times* said that my defeat was in many respects a victory because I had lasted so long and made Jansher work so hard. The *Daily Telegraph* reported that Jansher had rarely encountered such resistance. The great man himself was even more complimentary, saying: 'He can become world champion himself. He must keep working and concentrating. That's all.' Well, I was certainly prepared to do that.

Playing Jansher was a disorientating experience in a way. He was obviously in a different class from me at that time, but unlike with Jahingir it somehow didn't feel that way. I didn't come off court feeling that I had been blown away by someone totally out of my league. I had always felt that I was in the game. Looking back, I think the answer lies in Jansher's approach to squash, which was different from that of many other players. Someone like Jahingir would go all out to beat you as easily as possible. Jansher, by contrast, would play well within himself and just do enough to win. It gave you the impression that you always had a chance. In truth, however, if you did start to play better then Jansher would just go up a gear. Every time you stepped up, he stepped up too, and he always had that extra gear.

I was playing him regularly in the early '90s but he was way ahead of me at that time and usually beat me quite easily. By the summer of 1993, however, I was hoping that I could start to turn things around a little. I was getting better and stronger and was well established in the world top ten. It was time to make the next leap forward. That process was made easier by the fact that some of the top players from the previous decade were starting to fade. Jahingir had already gone and people like Chris Dittmar and Chris Robertson were bowing out.

Many of my contemporaries were pleased about this because they felt it would make it easier for them to get to the top. In my typically purist way, however, I felt exactly the opposite. I was disappointed to see them go because I had been looking forward to pitting my wits against them. I had beaten most of them, but not very often – I hadn't yet established a supremacy over them, which is what I had set out to do. I didn't want to replace them by default because they had retired. I wanted to replace them by outplaying them.

It wasn't to be, but I could still set my sights on Jansher. He was way out on his own with no one able to challenge him. I wanted to change that. My whole thinking at that time was how to find a game that was going to beat him. I knew that whatever happened, I would never beat him quickly. I didn't have the racket skills of someone like Rodney Martin who could pluck winning shots out of thin air and had an incredible capacity for getting the ball in the nick. Also, Jansher's ability to retrieve the ball meant the rallies would be kept going longer than against most opponents. I had to reconcile myself to long matches and that meant becoming as fit as possible. My training schedule was already as tough as anyone else's in the game, but I decided to step it up even more.

It was the summer of 1993. The season was over so it was a good time to get in some hard physical work in preparation for the coming campaign. My training sessions became more intense and I did more of them. It wasn't a ridiculous amount, but in hindsight it was probably too much. I may have set my target too high in attempting to match Jansher so quickly. In terms of both physical strength and skill I wasn't ready to challenge him at that time, yet that was what I was trying to do. It didn't occur to me that any of this might be damaging my health. I was completely focused on moving forward and, to be fair, I was enjoying spectacular success. I quickly got to number two in the world.

Jansher and I were pulling away from the rest and our matches were getting closer and closer. For a while I felt great. There was no hardship in competing against him. The only strain was working out how to beat him. I spent hours analysing his game, looking for weaknesses, and learnt a great deal about what I should and shouldn't do against him. For example, it used to be part of my game to play a lot of boasts, particularly off the backhand. I soon stopped doing that against him, though, because his incredible mobility about the court meant he would be on to the ball in a flash, ready to put me in trouble. Instead, I concentrated on upsetting his rhythm. He liked a slow steady game so I tried to step up the pace whenever possible by taking the ball early and forcing him to react more quickly than he liked. I also tried to develop my deceptive skills. If I could stop and start him, and make him unsure about what I was doing, then I might get him out of position. Even better, if I could get him going the wrong way then he might not recover in time to retrieve the ball. This was one of the strengths of my two-handed style – it was harder to read than orthodox techniques. It worked to a certain extent although, of course, the tactical battle swung both ways. He was learning about me as well, particularly the strengths and weaknesses of my two-handed approach. He played a lot of high shots to my forehand because he knew my style made it difficult for me to return them.

My carefully thought out tactics were fine in theory, but putting it all into practice was another matter entirely. It didn't help that Jansher changed his style a great deal during the years I played him. It was like trying to hit a moving target. As soon as you had him in your sights, he was gone. There were several reasons for this. In 1989, the rules were changed. The tin (the area at the bottom of the front wall where the ball is considered to be out) was lowered from 19 inches to 17. The idea was to encourage more exciting squash. A two-inch difference may not seem very significant, but it gave the advantage to people who played attacking shots. It's obviously easier to make a drop shot die at the front of the court if it only has to fall 17 inches instead of 19. This makes a big difference at professional level. The move coincided with the increasing use of glass courts to enable thousands of spectators to get a good view. They were erected in the middle of large arenas, and so tended to be cooler than the traditional brick-built courts. The slight drop in temperature made the ball less bouncy; it didn't sit up quite as much after someone had played a tight shot and was harder to retrieve. This, too, favoured the attacking player.

The changes coincided with the emergence of players like Martin, Dittmar and Robertson, who all favoured an attacking game. The change in the rules suited them and tipped the game a little in their favour. Players like Jansher, whose game was based primarily on defence, were put at a disadvantage. With the scales tipped in favour of the attackers, he would have to work much harder to stay with them. This would put a lot of pressure on his body and would take its toll very quickly. Maybe it's no coincidence that once the changes came in, Jahingir began to halt his run of defeats against Jansher and started chalking up some victories. Jansher understood the situation very quickly and realised he would have to change or risk being left behind.

To be fair, he responded magnificently. Before, he very rarely volleyed or stepped up the court to take the ball early. Now he started playing a variety of shots and putting the ball away at every opportunity. He quickly developed into one of the most skilful and attacking players of all time. His change in style made him more formidable than ever, because he retained his old strengths of superb court movement and retrieving power. As if all that wasn't enough, he was very good tactically as well and could change his game to suit the occasion. If there was a weakness in your game, you could be sure that he would find and exploit it for all it was worth.

I'm one of the few people still on the circuit who've played both Jahingir and Jansher, and you can probably guess one of the most frequent questions I'm asked: 'Which one of them was the best?' It's difficult to say, because they were both such great players. The statistics from their head-to-head matches don't tell us a great deal. Jansher won 19 games, while Jahingir won 18. If pressed, I would say that Jansher just shades it because of his incredible movement around the court and the way he was able to adapt his game. Towards the end of his career he wasn't as mobile as he had been as a teenager, but he made up for it with his improved racket skills. Jansher was the kind of player who didn't push himself any further than he needed to. I'm sure he had something in reserve even when he was winning all the time.

In spite of his increased prowess, I was getting steadily closer to him and started to pick up some titles. Thankfully for me, Jansher slipped up in the semi-final of the Portugese Open in 1993 and lost to Rodney Eyles. I seized the rare chance to win an event by beating Eyles in the final. My increased fitness was certainly helping me and, apart from Jansher, there were very few people who could beat me on a squash court when the going got tough. My next big battle against Jansher was in the final of the Qatar Open. I felt fine and took him to five games for the first time. That was probably some of the best squash I had ever played. I won the first and felt very strong. I continued to play well in the second and third games, but he just shaded it. I managed to find a little bit extra and took the fourth. I thought I was in with a great chance in the fifth game, but suddenly he just seemed to push a button and went up to a different level as he had done with so many players before. I was nowhere in it.

In spite of everything, however, those hard-to-define health problems refused to go away. I had felt fine in Qatar, but barely a week later, I started to feel groggy during the World Open in November 1993. Jansher got an easy 3–0 victory against me in the semi-final. That was disappointing because I had been in great form for a while, as I had shown at Qatar. Jonah Barrington came up to me after that game and asked what was wrong. He said I didn't seem quite right. I didn't really have an answer. I didn't have the flu, or anything I could describe, just felt generally a bit tired and jaded.

That feeling didn't last, so I didn't worry about it too much. In any case, the big games were coming round so quickly I hardly had time to think. Barely a month after losing so badly to Jansher in the World Open, I played him again, this time in the final of the World Super Series. It's an invitation tournament involving the top eight players in the world. I played well but he beat me 3–1. I had no complaints. He was still just that little bit too good for me. There were more epic battles in the early part of 1994: in March he beat me 3–1 in the final of the Portugese Open, and a month later he beat me by the same score as he had in the British Open, 3–1. I felt fine during all these matches and enjoyed every minute. I was still a long way off beating him but I could feel myself improving. If I could keep the same rate of progress up during the following season, then I might start to get some victories.

In June, however, I started to feel bad again. It was slightly worse this time than it had been before. I felt tired, struggled when I played, and didn't have as much energy as usual. I went to see my doctor, but he was quite relaxed about it; he just said I had probably been overdoing things a bit and needed to rest more. I had been resting anyway, but I decided to take things easy for another month. By August I felt better and stepped up my training again. This time it was a little up and down – some days I felt fine, others were a struggle.

Towards the end of August, I went to compete in the Hong Kong Open. I wasn't 100 per cent but I felt I could cope. I got through on determination more than anything else, and came up against Jansher in the semi-final. He was still too much for me and won 3–1. It's hard to describe how I felt. I wasn't exactly ill, but yet again I didn't feel quite right. I couldn't put my finger on the problem, and, as I wouldn't have known what to say was wrong with me, didn't say anything about it at the time. In any case, it would have seemed as though I was making excuses.

To add to the mystery, I felt great again within a few weeks – so much so that I got my first win over Jansher. I was playing for the German side OSC Ingolstadt in the final of the European club championships, while Jansher was playing for Squash Club de St Cloud in Paris. I beat him 3–0. It was only his second defeat of the year. Although victory in such a minor match was of limited significance, it gave me a great boost. I felt strong and was full of confidence as I went into the World Open in Barcelona a few weeks later. I was really on song during that period. I got through the early rounds quite easily, and beat Peter Nicol, who was rising towards the world's top five at that time, 3–1 in the semi-final.

Since it had become a professional tournament, no other English player had ever reached the final of the World Open. Just getting to the final was probably my biggest achievement at that point. It turned out to be a great match against Jansher, with both of us near the top of our form. I took the first game 9–5 and went ahead in the second. Everything was looking good, but then he began to reel me in and take the lead. Jansher took the game and continued to play brilliantly, winning 3–1. I have no complaints. I felt fine and was able to give it my best shot. Again, I came off court thinking 'What do I have to do to beat this man?' It was a question every top player was asking. Nevertheless, I had to accept that I had played well. Jansher acknowledged how close I was getting to him. He said afterwards: 'That was the best attack Peter has made on me. It shook me.'

Ironically, as I was stepping up my training and working harder, Jansher was doing exactly the opposite. As he got older and his game became more attacking, he eased up on his gruelling training routine. He obviously decided that his new style meant he didn't have to work as hard, and so there was no point in pushing his body and putting pressure on himself. He never liked to give anything away about his training schedules, but other Pakistani players confided that he was doing very little work in between tournaments. He would retreat to his beloved Peshawar and have long breaks doing nothing. Then, as the next event approached, he would start to prepare but would still only work three or four times a week, and even then it would be nothing like the tough sessions he put himself through when he was younger. He felt he had already built up a tremendous base strength and that was enough – he just wanted to keep it fine tuned without doing too much because he wanted to remain fresh.

The problem Jansher faced by locking himself away in Peshawar was the lack of top class opposition. Other players would meet up in their home countries to play practice matches, sometimes travelling hundreds of miles and staying away from home for days just to do some good quality work with people of a similar standard. There was no one of any real standard for Jansher to play in Peshawar, but he didn't seem to care. He played whoever was available and practised by himself. This, together with his relaxed approach to training, went against all conventional wisdom, but Jansher was always very much his own man. He learnt a lot from his brother and coach Mohibullah but was largely self-taught. I don't think he was the kind of character who would listen to anyone for very long.

His unorthodox approach extended to the way he arrived at tournaments. Most players would get there several days early to acclimatise to the local conditions, find their way around and start to make themselves comfortable. Jansher would often not turn up until the day he was playing, often just a few hours before the match was due to start. It was incredible. No one had adopted such a relaxed approach before. He would come straight from a 12-hour flight and walk onto court. People would shake their heads and say 'You can't work like that: you can't neglect training, play no one of any standard in practice then fly in at the last minute and expect to win.' With most players they would be right, but Jansher seemed to have no trouble coping. He would use the opening rounds to acclimatise and sharpen himself up and although he might look a little rusty at first, he would soon get back into it and be as formidable as ever. No one would have believed it possible had they not witnessed it. It took enormous confidence, of course; some would say arrogance. There were people who took it as a sign of disrespect for his fellow professionals, but I don't think that was the case – it was just the best preparation for him personally. He felt more relaxed staying back home in Peshawar and, as it worked, who's to say it was wrong?

Fortunately for him, he didn't have to endure a long flight to the tournament in which we had one of our best games ever, the final of the Pakistan Open. That was a great occasion, with the match played in front of one of the noisiest and most passionate crowds in the world. They had warmed a lot more to Jansher since the days when he upset them by having the audacity to beat Jahingir, but they still hadn't entirely taken him to their hearts. Jansher admitted later that he'd felt apprehensive before the game. He wasn't sure how the crowd would take to him and knew they didn't support him in the way they had other Pakistani champions. Yet he was representing their country, and so they wanted him to win. It was as if he had to fulfil their expectations without having their wholehearted support. I think that weighed heavily on him. He need not have worried. The crowd did cheer him on, but they weren't too hostile towards me either, which I appreciated. I doubt I would have got off so lightly if I'd been playing Jahingir.

During this period my health was again topsy-turvy. Only a few weeks earlier, I had played Jansher in the final of the Japan Open and not felt right at all. I lost 3–0 in a disappointingly one-sided match. By the time I met him in the final of the Pakistan Open, I felt fine again. It was puzzling, but I didn't have the time or the inclination to think about it much. I had to concentrate on the game.

It turned out to be a classic. One of the best matches I have ever played in. I took the first game and went ahead 14–12 in the second. This was a fantastic opportunity for me. If Jansher had a weakness, it was a tendency to get downhearted if he fell behind. It was rare for him to go 2–0 down, and I hoped that if I could get him there his spirits would sink and he wouldn't try so hard. It was a good theory, but putting it into practice was the problem. He pulled the game back to 14–14 but I still fancied my chances. Then, in the deciding rally, I had a stroke called against me. I'm biased obviously, but I didn't agree that it was a stroke and it was very frustrating to lose the game. It would have brought a tremendous advantage. This threw me off balance for a while and I lost the third game, but pulled myself back together and won the fourth comfortably. It was poised for a tense finish, but Jansher showed his class by again stepping up a gear and taking it comfortably. He'd done me yet again.

It was a brutal game physically, but then that's squash at the top level. I think the crowd enjoyed it. Many Pakistani fans came up afterwards to congratulate me on my performance and commiserate with me for having lost. Some said they were hoping I would win, which suggests that Jansher still wasn't as popular as Jahingir.

I'd been fine during the tournament, but afterwards I started to feel tired and listless again. Again, I went to see my doctor and again he said there was nothing wrong with me. He was quite casual about it and told me to take a few weeks off and rest. I insisted that I was sure there was something seriously wrong with me, but the doctor was adamant that I was fine. He even said that if I was able to play squash I couldn't be very ill. I wasn't satisfied with this. The fact that I was able to carry on playing owed more to willpower than to good health. Sometimes I felt terrible. I asked to see a specialist. He was reluctant to refer me but I was determined. Eventually, he agreed and I went to have some blood tests done. They didn't reveal anything conclusive, so it was back to resting again. By now, I was starting to worry. The uncertainty of not knowing what was wrong made things worse.

I rested for a few weeks, but it didn't seem to make any difference to my health. Sometimes I felt fine; at other times, I felt increasingly listless. It was hard to know what to do, but in the absence of any definite diagnosis I felt I was left with little choice but to press on. I pulled myself together and played the Portuguese Open. I knew I was far from right but I still managed to get to the final. My determination drove me on. Sadly, that wasn't enough against someone like Jansher and he beat me quite easily again. By now, there were times when I was starting to feel disturbingly ill.

In 1995 I took most of January and February off, but it didn't seem to make much difference. I started seeing more doctors but they seemed as bemused as me. Some were sceptical, others were very sympathetic, but none of them seemed to have much idea what to say other than to rest. As

I was feeling increasingly tired, that seemed obvious and I was already doing it anyway. I was disappointed, not only with their inability to help but also with their lack of concern. It wasn't very encouraging. I felt I had little option but to pull myself together and get on with things.

That's precisely what I did as March approached, bringing the British Open, the biggest tournament in the game. I went into it full of hope that I could do well, only to suffer the most crushing and humiliating defeat of my career. After that 3–0 mauling by Jansher, when every movement on court required a huge act of will, I could no longer put worries about my health to the back of my mind. Something serious was wrong and I would have to face it head on.

I saw more doctors and rested for several months. Then it occurred to me that the symptoms were similar to those I had when I had glandular fever. There were the swollen glands, the flu-like feeling, the lack of energy and sense of listlessness. Perhaps the fever had returned. I went back to the doctor and had more tests done. They came back negative: I wasn't suffering from glandular fever, although I still had the anti-bodies in my system. In a way, I was disappointed that it wasn't a recurrence of my earlier illness. At least I would have known what it was and how to deal with it. I was now racked with uncertainty and that was becoming a problem in itself.

A friend, the squash player Jason Nicolle, told me of a naturopath and nutritionist called Mike Ash who had dealt with people suffering from symptoms of fatigue. He lived all the way down in Devon, but I decided to see if he could help me. He did some tests and decided that my liver might not be working properly. This rang true; I remembered the stabbing pains I had been feeling in the area of my liver shortly after the British Open final. Mr Ash put me on an exclusion detoxification diet to give my liver time to rest. I couldn't eat red meat, fried food, anything with additives or preservatives, tea or coffee. I also wasn't allowed bread because it was thought I might have a wheat allergy. Instead, I was to concentrate on wholesome food like rice, potatoes and vegetables. He told me to stick to the diet for two months, stop all my training and get plenty of rest. When I returned two months later, he did some more tests and my liver was fine. I was allowed to start training again. Unfortunately, nothing had changed. I still felt weak.

Then one morning in June I opened a hospital letter that upped the stakes to a far more worrying level. A few weeks before the start of the British Open, my doctor had sent me to Kettering Hospital to have a series of tests done. The results showed that my muscle enzyme level was grossly high. The doctors there thought I might have a muscle wasting disease. Those words sent a chill right through me. The letter recommended that I see a neurologist for further treatment. I read the letter several times. The interruption to my career now seemed secondary; I was far more concerned about the threat to my general health. I had several anxious days waiting for an appointment at my local hospital, the Queen's Medical Centre. I turned up, full of trepidation, but it turned out to be a false alarm. The specialist assured me that athletes often get high readings in enzyme tests and it was nothing to worry about.

It was a tremendous relief, but also strangely frustrating because again I was back to square one. It was now the middle of the summer and I hadn't played since the British Open. I had been resting for four months, but still wasn't feeling right. I had to work out what to do, but it was hard because no one knew what was wrong. There was no advice available. Part of me was saying I should rest, but another part was saying I had tried that and it hadn't done any good. I might as well start training again and see what happened.

I did some easy work for a few weeks and then decided to do a harder session just to see how I would get on. It was only for about half an hour, and wasn't a particularly tough session by my usual standards. Nevertheless, I found it difficult and was very tired. Afterwards I went to bed and slept for about 14 hours. When I woke up the next morning, I felt terrible. It felt as though every muscle and bone in my body was stiff and aching. It was hard to understand. Only six months earlier I was one of the fittest athletes in the world. It was very deflating, and made me realise even more that something very serious was going on inside me.

All the time I was aware that I was losing ground. Before the British Open, I had been challenging to become the world number one. Now I was missing tournaments and starting to slip down the rankings. I found that very hard to bear. Most athletes get a bit paranoid when they're missing training: you can't escape the fear that other people are pulling ahead of you. The debate went on in my mind for several weeks. Train or rest? In the end, I decided to start training again. It seemed more positive to face the problem head on and actively do something about it rather than sit waiting passively for an improvement that might never come.

I gradually built up my training, and was pleasantly surprised when I didn't feel too bad. Perhaps I would be able to get going again. In September, I went to Japan to play my first tournament in six months. I lost in the first round to Mark Chaloner. I was amazed and disturbed by how much ground I had lost in that seemingly short time. Mark was ranked about 25 in the world, and I would normally expect to beat him without too much trouble. Now he was the one chalking up an easy 3–0 victory. For most of the game I was a yard off the pace, and felt like I was chasing shadows. I told myself that maybe it was a one-off. I would be all right when I got match fit again and had time to re-acclimatise to the pace of the game at the top level. There were no major tournaments for another month, so I only had to play one-off league matches. I couldn't even manage those. After a few games I started to feel terrible again and ended up in bed with flu – or what seemed like flu – for the second time in six months, making it even more depressing.

I was still consulting different doctors in the hope of making a breakthrough. My manager sent me to a specialist in London who did some tests and decided I had a throat infection. This was no doubt true, but it was coincidental, not the main cause of my problem. My fatigue symptoms persisted long after my throat started to feel better.

After a while, I went to see Mike Ash again. He had been studying some new research from America, which suggested that it was possible for the adrenaline glands to stop functioning. This affected the endocrine system and caused a fatigue problem. I was quite excited by this and thought that perhaps it could be a significant breakthrough. Mr Ash made no promises but thought it would be worth a try. He gave me some herbal tablets to boost the adrenaline system and I took them feeling reasonably optimistic. It was no good. The tablets made me feel worse. I persevered with them for about a month but then gave up.

By now, it was nearly Christmas. I was confused and unsure about what to do next. Then I went to see a student friend who was doing a sports science degree. She had a magazine called *Peak Performance* which contained an article about a swimmer suffering from something called chronic fatigue syndrome. I had never heard of it. I started reading the piece quite casually, but became more and more interested as the symptoms this swimmer had suffered seemed remarkably like the ones I had been experiencing. He had been out for 18 months but was now back training again. At the end of the article, it gave the name of the man who had helped him overcome the problem. His name was Dr Richard Budgett, a former athlete who worked at the Olympic Training Centre. I read the article again and made a note of the doctor's name. I felt a rush of excitement and anticipation. Might this man be able to help me?

# 6

# ILL? BUT YOU DON'T LOOK ILL!

There are probably times in all our lives when we just want to hand over control to someone else. Let them make the decisions, let them take the responsibility. It leaves us free to relax, switch off and hopefully recover. We can do this safe in the knowledge that no one can accuse us of slacking. We're simply following instructions. That's the state I had reached by the time I went to see Dr Budgett. I was mentally and physically drained. Even reading a book could leave me exhausted. After more than a year of fighting something I didn't understand, I had no energy left for anything.

At that point, I was certainly ready to hand over responsibility. There was something within me that desperately wanted to rest, but I wasn't able to do it. I thought that maybe I was being lazy. Deep down I knew that wasn't the case, but I still had doubts. There was always part of me saying I should shake it off and push myself harder, because until then no one had been able to tell me what was happening.

I went to see Dr Budgett at the British Olympic Medical Centre in London. He asked me to describe my symptoms. I told I always felt exhausted and that my muscles got very tired during exercise. They were heavy, sore and could take days to recover. I was sleeping all the time, yet not feeling refreshed. My concentration wasn't very good and it was hard to find the drive to do anything. Dr Budgett then asked about other symptoms. Had there been times when I had swollen glands and a sore throat? Was there a lack of appetite? Had there been occasions when I had felt depressed? I said yes, I had experienced all those symptoms at different times. He asked me about my medical history. I told him there had been lots of periods over the last few years when I had felt unwell without being able to say exactly what was wrong. I mentioned that I'd had glandular fever. He said that was very significant. Then he told me that I was suffering from chronic fatigue syndrome (CFS). My symptoms were typical of the illness, and so was my medical background: many sufferers have previously suffered from viral infections such as glandular fever.

I sat back to take it all in. It was the first time anyone had put a name to my problem, and that was a relief in itself. Suffering from an illness that couldn't be defined or explained had given it all an air of unreality, as if there wasn't really anything wrong with me at all. I had been beginning to fear it was all in my head, as none of the doctors I had been to see previously had been able to find anything wrong. I later discovered that this is a common feeling among CFS sufferers in the early stages, before the illness is diagnosed. It felt good to know that I wasn't alone; other people experienced the same problems.

I was comforted by being able to say what was wrong with me, but I wanted to know more. What exactly was chronic fatigue syndrome? Dr Budgett was one of the leading authorities on the illness, yet he was very honest in admitting that there was no one definite cause and certainly no one definite cure. He felt that I had probably pushed myself too hard after coming back from my bout of glandular fever. The problem was then made worse as I continued to push forward with my career. He said my heavy workload of playing and training, together with the stresses of competing and travelling, added to the problem. It would be necessary to remove those stresses in order to recover.

I listened to what he had to say with great interest. For the first time, I felt that someone really understood my problem. I wasn't always convinced that some of the other doctors I had seen were on the right track. I always did what they said because I wanted to recover but I didn't have that much confidence that it would work. Dr Budgett's diagnosis, however, felt right because it was much closer to the feelings I had been experiencing. One of the first questions I asked was how long it would be before I could play again. He told me it would be nine months to a year – an awful long time, but I knew I would have to accept it. He told me he had seen people who were far worse than I was and they had managed to recover. I found that very reassuring.

Dr Budgett drew up a programme of what I should do to get better. The most important thing was to get plenty of rest. However, he didn't advocate

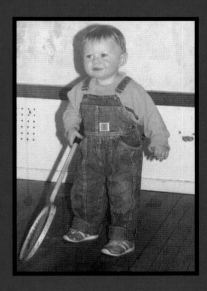
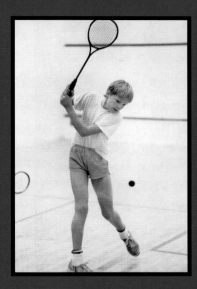

ABOVE LEFT: EARLY STARTER. I LOVED PLAYING SQUASH FROM THE FIRST TIME I PICKED
UP A RACKET AT MY FAMILY'S CLUB AT KEGWORTH IN LEICESTERSHIRE.

ABOVE RIGHT: I WAS TOO SMALL TO HOLD THE RACKET WITH ONE
HAND WHEN I STARTED PLAYING SO I USED TWO. SEVERAL COACHES
TRIED TO MAKE ME CHANGE, BUT THE STYLE STUCK.

BELOW: PLAYING SIMON PARKE IN THE FINAL OF THE BRITISH UNDER-14S NATIONAL
CHAMPIONSHIPS. WE'VE BEEN SLUGGING IT OUT ON SQUASH COURTS ALL OVER THE
WORLD EVER SINCE AND HAVE BECOME GOOD FRIENDS.

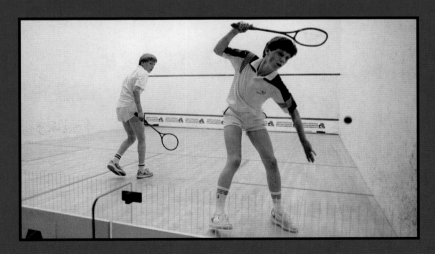

RIGHT: BEATING PETER NICOL
TO BECOME
BRITISH NATIONAL CHAMPION
IN 1994.

BELOW: JONAH BARRINGTON
HAS BEEN ONE OF THE
BIGGEST NAMES IN SQUASH
FOR OVER 30 YEARS. HE'S
BEEN A BIG INSPIRATION
SINCE HE COACHED
ME AS A CHILD.

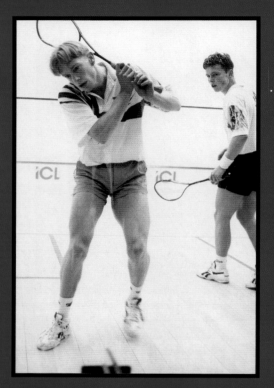

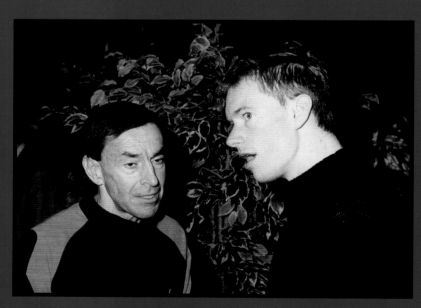

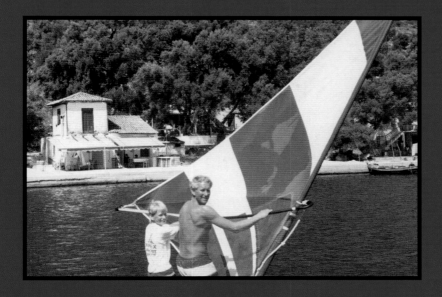

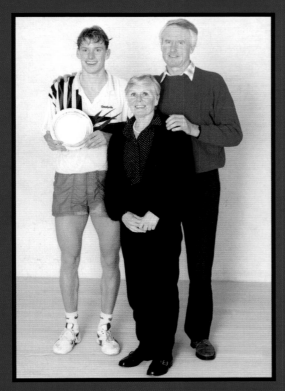

ABOVE: WINDSURFING
WITH DAD.

LEFT: WITH MY MUM AND
DAD AFTER BECOMING
BRITISH NATIONAL
CHAMPION. THEY ALWAYS
ENCOURAGED ME WHEN I
WAS YOUNGER, BUT
NEVER PUT ANY PRESSURE
ON ME AS SOME PARENTS
DID WITH THEIR
CHILDREN.

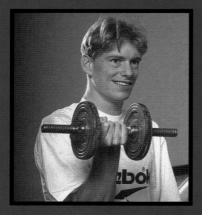

BEFORE I BECAME ILL I WAS ONE OF
THE FITTEST SPORTSMEN IN THE
WORLD AND REGULARLY
PUT MYSELF THROUGH LONG,
GRUELLING TRAINING SESSIONS. I NO
LONGER FEEL IT'S NECESSARY TO
TRAIN THAT HARD.

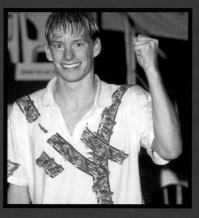

JOY AFTER CLAIMING JAHINGIR'S SCALP.
I WAS ONE OF ONLY FIVE PEOPLE TO
BEAT HIM THROUGHOUT HIS INCREDIBLE
CAREER.

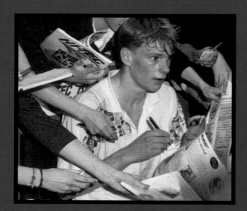

BIG EVENTS IN SQUASH TEND TO BE VERY
RELAXED COMPARED WITH OTHER SPORTS.
IT'S EASY FOR THE FANS TO MEET THE
PLAYERS, WHICH MAKES FOR A FRIENDLY
ATMOSPHERE — UNTIL WE GET ON COURT, OF
COURSE!

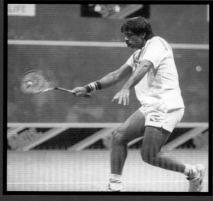

THE LEGENDARY JAHINGIR KHAN WAS ONE
OF MY BOYHOOD HEROES AND BROKE ALL
THE RECORDS. HE WENT FIVE-AND-A-HALF
YEARS UNBEATEN IN THE 1980S. WHEN I
TURNED PROFESSIONAL, I HAD TO FORGET
ABOUT HIS HERO STATUS AND TREAT HIM
AS JUST ANOTHER PLAYER.

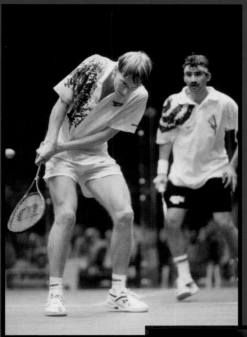

PLAYING JANSHER KHAN IN THE FINAL OF THE 1995 BRITISH OPEN. MY ILLNESS MEANT I HAD NO ENERGY TO COMPETE. IT WAS THE WORST PERFORMANCE OF MY LIFE AND MADE ME REALISE SOMETHING WAS SERIOUSLY WRONG.

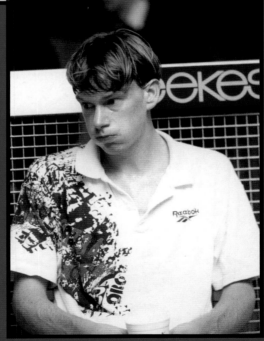

BEWILDERED AND EXHAUSTED WITH NOWHERE TO HIDE. I COULD FEEL A THOUSAND PAIRS OF EYES BURNING INTO ME:  WHY HAD I PLAYED SO BADLY?

BEATING JONATHAN POWER IN THE
WORLD OPEN DURING MY BRIEF
COMEBACK ATTEMPT IN 1997. IT
WAS ONE OF MY BEST
PERFORMANCES, CONSIDERING
THAT I WAS STARTING TO FEEL ILL
AGAIN.

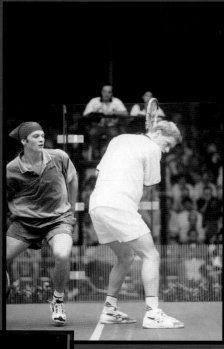

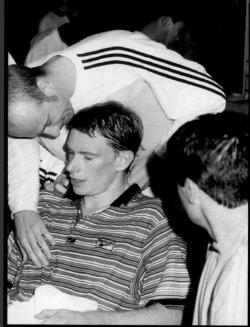

THE GAME AGAINST POWER
TOOK TOO MUCH OUT OF ME.
I HAD GOT THROUGH ON
ADRENALINE AND
DETERMINATION.

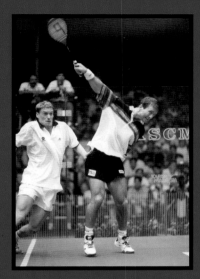

RODNEY EYLES AT FULL STRETCH. HE WAS MY SEMI-FINAL OPPONENT AFTER I BEAT POWER. SADLY, I WASN'T STRONG ENOUGH AND LOST EASILY. EYLES WAS IN GREAT FORM AND WENT ON TO BE WORLD CHAMPION.

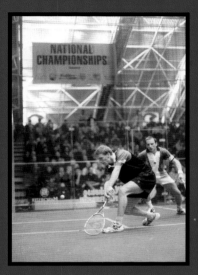

TWO MARATHON FIVE-SET VICTORIES OVER PAUL JOHNSON IN THE TOURNAMENT OF CHAMPIONS AND THE BRITISH NATIONAL CHAMPIONSHIPS CONVINCED ME I COULD STILL FIND THE ENERGY TO COMPETE AT THE TOP LEVEL.

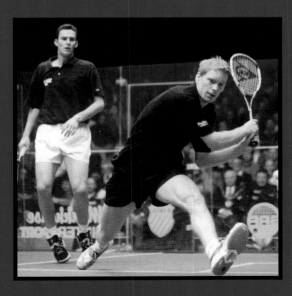

ROLLING BACK THE YEARS. IN BEATING DAVID EVANS TO BECOME BRITISH CHAMPION, I RECAPTURED SOME OF THE STRENGTH AND FORM I ENJOYED BEFORE I BECAME ILL. IT WAS A WONDERFUL FEELING.

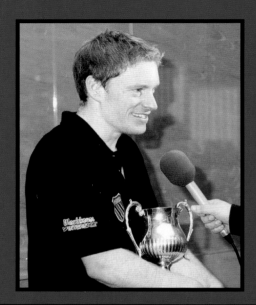

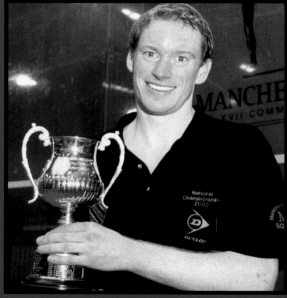

TOP AND ABOVE: BACK IN THE LIMELIGHT. I GOT A TREMENDOUS
RESPONSE FROM THE FANS, THE MEDIA AND EVERYONE
INVOLVED IN SQUASH WHEN I BECAME BRITISH NATIONAL CHAMPION
AFTER FOUR YEARS OUT OF THE GAME. IT MADE
ME REALISE HOW MUCH I HAD BEEN MISSING.

doing nothing at all – that would mean my body could become weak and out of shape. Initially, the plan was to do about 15 minutes of gentle exercise a day, nothing more strenuous than walking or an easy session on a bike. I was to wear a heart monitor and not let my heart rate get above 120/130 beats per minute – quite low when you're exercising, but anything more would have left me feeling drained. He also urged me to take care with my diet and cut out foods like sugar and caffeine, which the body had to work hard to remove. I had to get plenty of sleep, go to bed at regular times and try not to worry about things. It was important to remove all stress.

My meeting with Dr Budgett gave me a tremendous boost because at last I felt I was getting somewhere. At first it was disappointing that it would take a year to get better, but I soon got used to the idea. It was just such a great relief for it all to be explained, and to at last have a definite plan of what I was going to do. I went home feeling very positive. It was exciting to think that at last I could start to move forward.

My family and friends were all very helpful and sympathetic when I told them I was suffering from CFS. I soon discovered, however, that not everyone was so understanding. CFS was very controversial at that time; some people didn't regard it as a genuine illness. Indeed, many doctors didn't believe it existed at all; an attitude that caused widespread anger and resentment among sufferers. Many felt they were being treated as malingerers when in fact they were seriously ill. It was like adding insult to injury. This was brought home to me when I watched a TV discussion programme on the subject. The presenter, Esther Rantzen, did her best to keep things calm, but the audience started booing a doctor who seemed to suggest that CFS was largely psychological and that many patients had shown significant improvements when treated with anti-depressants. This outraged the sufferers, who made it clear that they were tired of being told the problem was psychological. I could understand their frustration. Having experienced how debilitating it could be, I wouldn't like to be told it was all in the mind either. Many people in the audience were either sufferers themselves or related to someone who had the illness, including Esther Rantzen. Her 18-year-old daughter Emily was seriously ill at that time. Emily was very sensitive to noise and light, suffered from severe headaches and, like all victims, was prey to debilitating muscular fatigue. At times, she was so weak that she needed to use a wheelchair.

This television talk show wasn't my first introduction to the debate raging among doctors and sufferers about the causes of CFS, but it was certainly the most dramatic. There was real anger on the faces of the people in the audience, but when you consider the amount of negative publicity CFS had received at that time it's hardly surprising. The illness first eased its way into public consciousness in the '80s when the tabloid press dismissed it as 'yuppie flu', a label that made for easy headlines but unfortunately made many people take the illness less seriously, in the same way that the label of 'gay plague' lessened the impact of Aids. People who didn't consider themselves to be yuppies, which was just about everyone, thought the illness would never affect them.

To be fair, though, until I received the diagnosis from Dr Budgett I was as ignorant as everyone else about CFS. If I had heard about it at all, it was in the context of alarmist and dubious reports in the press, only half read and quickly forgotten. Now my attitude was, of course, going to change. I wanted to know as much as possible about the illness that had been turning my life upside down for nearly two years. I armed myself with as many books, articles and information leaflets as I could find. The results were surprising. Far from being an invention of the 1980s, this was an illness with a long and dramatic history. Noel Coward, Charles Darwin and Florence Nightingale all suffered from CFS, although it had only recently acquired that title. For hundreds of years it went under an array of vague names such as 'the vapours' or 'the fever'. It also had more impressive sounding medical names such as 'febricula', meaning little fever, or 'neurasthenia', relating to weakness in the nervous system. By the 1950s it was being called 'chronic brucellosis' and then 'fibromyalgia'.

Much of my information at this time came from a book called *Living with ME* by Dr Charles Shepherd. He was the Medical Director to the ME Association and, as a sufferer himself, was better placed than most people to understand the problems. As I read of the scepticism of some doctors, I saw how the press might have been encouraged to come up with the term 'yuppie flu'. If large sections of the medical profession didn't take the illness seriously, why should the headline writers? And I realised that it was hardly surprising that the doctors who treated the likes of Charles Darwin and Florence Nightingale could not agree on a name. The modern medical profession was doing no better.

The disease had a different name in virtually every country in the world, and in some places it went under several names at the same time. The Icelandic people called it 'Icelandic disease' as if it belonged only to them. To New Zealanders it was 'Tapanui flu'. In America it had gone under a variety of titles such as 'epidemic neuromyasthenia' and eventually 'chronic fatigue syndrome' and 'immune dysfunction syndrome'. The most dramatic was the name given to it by the Japanese, 'low natural killer cell syndrome'.

I read through Dr Shepherd's book and saw that about 70 per cent of CFS patients had previously suffered what was called a precipitating illness. This was usually some sort of infection which would eventually clear up but leave the patient weakened and susceptible to CFS. These infections could be things like flu, gastroenteritis or tonsillitis. In my case it was glandular fever, as Dr Budgett had pointed out.

Glandular fever is caused by the Epstein-Barr virus, which also causes other infections. Many sufferers of CFS have been infected with the virus. In fact, it has become so closely associated with CFS that one of the early names for the disease in America was chronic Epstein-Barr viral disease. I discovered that once you're infected with EBV it stays in your system for life, but doesn't normally cause any harm as it's kept under control by natural killer cells which form part of the immune system. However, a few American doctors formulated a theory that the EBV might be somehow reactivated to create fatigue-like symptoms. This could only happen if the immune system wasn't working properly, probably because the natural killer cells weren't functioning as normal. This would tie in with the Japanese name for the disease, low natural killer cell syndrome.

Could it be that there was something lacking in my body's ability to fight illness? The Americans called the illness chronic fatigue and immune dysfunction syndrome. Could there be something wrong with my immune system? Nothing was showing up in blood tests, but what did that prove? Perhaps the necessary blood test hadn't yet been developed. I remembered the number of times I had had flu and colds over the previous few years. It was very interesting to speculate, but it didn't really take me anywhere. The more I looked at it, the more I could see theories that seemed reasonable but couldn't be proved or disproved. No one could tell one way or another. It was very frustrating, so I tried to put it out of my mind.

There was nothing I could do but follow the advice of the doctors. I tried to settle down to what for me was a very unusual life of resting and relaxing. I also tried to eat as well as possible and get lots of sleep. After the traumas of the previous two years, it was a great relief not to have to think about training and having to push myself when I really didn't have the energy. I just wanted to do whatever the doctor said. To have him tell me I must rest was a tremendous relief. It was what I wanted, and now it had been officially sanctioned.

After about three months, I went back to see Dr Budgett. I told him I was still feeling unwell but had done the 15 minutes a day exercising without any problem. That was positive and he said I could increase it a little. I went back home and started exercising for 30 minutes a day. It was still very gentle, and again I coped with it quite easily. The excitement I had felt after first seeing Dr Budgett was starting to fade, however. I was feeling better but it was only a small improvement. Time was ticking by and I still had the same symptoms.

Another few months passed without any real progress being made. I went back to see Dr Budgett and upped my training a little more, which was fine, but mentally things started to get on top of me. I was still feeling bad, day in day out, and that was starting to bring me down. Allowing myself to become excited about the prospect of getting better was probably counter-productive, because when the recovery showed no sign of happening I began to lose faith a little. Nevertheless, there was little I could do except keep following the advice of the experts and try to stick to Dr Budgett's instructions about resting and reducing stress.

The concept of not worrying was very difficult, however. I couldn't help but be concerned about when I would be able to play again or, indeed, whether I would ever play again. I continued to find out more about CFS and its history. I was amazed at how widespread it is, affecting millions of people all over the world. Usually the cases are isolated, but there have also been several well-documented outbreaks producing hundreds of sufferers in closely defined locations. These have quite often been hospitals: 200 members of staff were hit by an outbreak at the Los Angeles County General Hospital in 1934. They complained of tiredness, muscle fatigue and generally feeling unwell. Many smaller outbreaks followed in other parts of the United States. The most famous was at Lake

Tahoe in Nevada, and attracted a lot of media attention, because the lake was an expensive holiday area for the well-off. The sight of so many high rollers going down with this strange affliction made for an interesting story. Many of them were middle-class professionals, which may have contributed to the illness becoming known as yuppie flu.

England had similar experiences. The most prominent was at the Royal Free Hospital in London in 1955. People from all over the city's northern suburbs started complaining of flu-like symptoms with sore throats, fever, swollen glands and dizziness. The details varied slightly from patient to patient but one problem common to all of them was that even the slightest bit of exercise could leave their muscles feeling exhausted. There were more than 200 cases. Doctors ran the usual tests, but couldn't find anything wrong. They were baffled. Something was happening, but they had no idea what.

Worse was to come. Over the next few months, many of those same doctors as well as many nurses developed similar symptoms themselves. In less than two weeks, 70 medical staff were taken ill. They started to show the same symptoms as the patients they had been treating in the previous few months. There was obviously some sort of infection being spread, but what was it? Nobody knew. Whatever the cause, the effect was so bad that the hospital had to close due to lack of staff. This obviously attracted a lot of press attention; it's not every day a hospital has to close because of some mystery illness.

For want of a better name, the condition became known as the Royal Free disease. Most of the patients and staff eventually recovered, at least partially, but many remained permanently ill. A consultant at the Royal's infectious diseases unit, Dr Melvin Ramsay, was struck by the way that so many of his colleagues, men and women who were highly dedicated and previously very fit and healthy, had succumbed to this strange affliction. He began a lifetime study to discover more about it. Ramsay was the one who came up with the name by which the disease was to be known until well into the 1990s, myalgic encephalomyelitis; ME for short. Myalgic refers to the muscle pain, and encephalomyelitis suggests that it's caused by an inflammation in the brain and the nervous system.

The disease remained controversial for years, with many doctors refusing to believe it existed. Then, in October 1996, doctors from the three royal colleges representing physicians, psychiatrists and GPs published their findings from a long and exhaustive investigation into the illness. Their work was based on 250 research papers and case studies. They concluded that what they had found was a serious and life-affecting illness that could and should be treated. The report estimated that between 1 and 2.6 per cent of the population was affected by it at some stage. This meant there could be somewhere in the region of a million sufferers in Britain alone. The report said that the term 'myalgic encephalomyelitis' should no longer be used, because although the experts weren't sure of the precise cause, they were confident that it was not due to any inflammation of the brain or nervous system as the name encephalomyelitis suggested. They preferred to call it chronic fatigue syndrome.

The investigation by the three colleges had been commissioned by the government's chief medical officer at the time, Sir Kenneth Calman. Even so, it wasn't until two years later in 1998, after much campaigning by sufferers and their supporters, that CFS was given official recognition by the Department of Health. On 16 July, Sir Kenneth finally provided the acknowledgement that people had been waiting for when he said: 'I recognise that ME is a real entity. It is distressing and debilitating. It affects a large number of people and poses a significant challenge to the medical profession.'

Sir Kenneth also announced that he was convening a special committee to develop methods of clinical practice and the management of chronic fatigue syndrome. He insisted that care should be provided by the National Health Service and urged doctors to establish good relationships with sufferers as a basis of good medicine. It may seem incredible now that doctors should ever have to be encouraged to develop a good relationship with their patients, but that's a measure of how chronic fatigue syndrome was perceived by many people at that time. Thankfully, the climate was changing, as was made clear by comments from Alan McGregor, a professor of medicine at King's College Hospital, London: 'The idea that this is a disease of so-called yuppies is completely erroneous. This is a disease that can affect anyone. Social background is irrelevant. We're not in any doubt that this is a substantial burden of ill-health in the community.'

Professor MacGregor acknowledged that CFS had been subjected to 'enormous ignorance and scepticism'. When asked about the work of the new committee he said: 'Patients want better diagnosis and better tests. They want to be taken seriously by their doctors and they want their doctors to be well informed.' Sadly, as I sat reading up on CFS back in 1996, this kind of enlightenment was still two years away. The controversy was still raging and that's what led to the kind of outbursts seen on the Esther Rantzen programme.

As a newly diagnosed sufferer, I was approaching the subject with an open mind. Having experienced such debilitating weakness in my muscles and other highly tangible symptoms such as swollen glands, I was in no doubt that my illness had a physical basis. However, I was prepared to accept that there might have been psychological characteristics that pre-disposed me towards being a sufferer. The doctors who drew up the report of chronic fatigue syndrome commissioned by Sir Kenneth Calman concluded that in most cases there were both physical and psychological elements to the problem. Dr Robert Kendall, president of the Royal College of Psychiatrists, said: 'To try to distinguish between a physical illness and a psychological one is not just wrong, it's meaningless.'

This struck me as a sensible approach as I couldn't see how physical and mental wellbeing could ever be regarded as two separate entities. They were intertwined no matter what the illness happened to be. I had seen people suffering from all sorts of ailments and injuries, whether it be a minor cold or something more traumatic like a broken leg. It seemed obvious to me that in all cases the person's state of mind will have an influence on the extent to which they allow their condition to affect their lives and how well they recover. However, the difference between CFS and things like broken legs is that people can see when a bone is fractured. They'll understand that the man in the plaster cast is feeling down because his condition is laying him low. No one will imagine that the broken leg is something simply brought on because the man needs to pull himself together. The CFS sufferer is less fortunate. There's no X-ray showing a broken bone, no blood test showing up some abnormality. Consequently, CFS sufferers who are depressed by their condition aren't given the same leeway as the man with the broken leg. It's all too easy for sceptics to say the problem is all in the mind, and that the feeling of fatigue is brought on by a depressed state of mind rather than the other way round. This attitude seems ridiculous but it's the way some people reacted.

Faced with such wildly differing opinions, there could be no certainty about anything and I must admit there were times throughout my illness when I doubted myself. I had strange thoughts that maybe I was making it up and wasn't ill at all. I questioned myself and my motives, wondered if everything was as bad as I thought. Maybe I should be able to pull myself together, as the sceptics suggested. Thoughts like these could catch me unawares. I wasn't aware of it at the time, but friends told me afterwards that there were periods when I did seem very down and depressed.

On one level I had no doubt that I was suffering from a real illness. On another, I think I was influenced by people who dismissed it as something purely psychological. No one can be 100 per cent certain of their own make-up and motivations. When you're faced by so many conflicting opinions, you're bound to have doubts about how well you know yourself. I'm sure these thoughts have haunted many people suffering from CFS, some of whom are much worse off than I was. I knew of people who were confined to bed permanently. It must have been terrible for them to be told there was nothing wrong with them. I heard of others who forced themselves to start working too early because they were told the problem was all in their head. They ended up making themselves worse.

There were times when I wished it *were* all in the mind; if it had been I'm sure I would have been able to deal with it. My willpower had always been one of my strongest assets. I understood the relationship between my mind and body very well. I knew when I could force myself beyond the limits of my physical capability, as I had done in countless matches. But I also knew what it was like to ask my body to perform and get no response at all. I recalled those days after playing Jansher Khan when I felt exhausted. I remembered how I tried to will those aching limbs to stand, to move and to run. They couldn't do it. There was nothing there, no strength at all. I knew that wasn't something that could be dismissed as being simply in my mind. It was real; it was physical. Having said that, I had no particular axe to grind. I just wanted to get better. If someone could have demonstrated to me that the problem was psychological, I would have felt no shame in that. Instead, I would have rushed to ask them to explain it to me fully. 'So, what is going on my mind? Where's the problem? Tell me what's wrong and I'll fix it.' No one could do such a thing, obviously.

After about six months, I was feeling better but was still nowhere near ready to start training properly again. I continued seeing Dr Budgett and was getting advice on diet from Mike Ash in Devon. I was satisfied with the treatment they were giving me but was always looking around for ideas from other people who might be able to help. As there were so many conflicting opinions about CFS and its treatment, it seemed wise to keep all options open. I had joined a CFS group by this time and started getting a newsletter from them. One article contained information about Dr Lucinda Scott at St Bartholomew's Hospital in London. She had been having some success with patients so I went to see her. She prescribed an anti-depressant drug called Sertraline that had helped people with similar symptoms to mine. I tried it, but unfortunately it had no effect. It was very disappointing. I was back where I had started.

Reassuringly, Dr Scott agreed with Dr Budgett and Mr Ash that I should get plenty of rest and continue to build up my training programme very gradually. However, there were other doctors writing articles in CFS newsletters insisting that total rest was the answer and that sufferers shouldn't attempt any work or exercise at all. Other doctors went to the opposite extreme, saying that sufferers should ignore the problem and carry on working as if nothing had happened. If they did this, they would eventually recover and get back to normal.

Looking back, I realised I had tried all three approaches towards rest and exercise. Before seeing Dr Budgett, I had tried total rest for three or four months without getting any better. I had also attempted to battle through the problem by continuing to play and train, but that hadn't worked for me either. Now I was trying to build up gradually. I was feeling better, but was still a long way from being right. I was beginning to wonder if anything would work. It was all very confusing but I decided to stick to the gradual approach. It seemed to make more sense than going to extremes.

At this point, squash was very much taking a secondary role in my life. I wanted to play again, of course, but foremost in my mind was my general health. I wanted to wake up not feeling tired and drained of energy all the time. One of the hardest things was explaining to people what was wrong with me. My parents had always been good at listening, but it was very complex: it was difficult for me to describe, and so it was obviously difficult for them to understand. It was very frustrating for them because as parents they wanted to help. They had always been able to advise me in the past but they didn't know anything about this, so there was little they could do but offer moral support.

It was even more difficult explaining my condition to people who weren't so sympathetic. The reaction I used to get from people was: 'Ill? You don't look ill. You look really well.' They meant no harm and were probably just trying to make me feel better, but it's one of the most annoying things people can say to someone suffering from CFS. It comes across as if they're saying: 'You look okay so you must be okay.' Nothing could be further from the truth. There might have been some people who thought I was just opting out or something like that, but I didn't care. I knew the truth and so did people close to me. My family and close friends all knew how much my career meant to me, and that there was no way I would stop playing unless I had to.

Because I was a sportsman, it was probably a lot easier for me than for many other sufferers. People could look at me and see that I had pushed myself physically for several years. It made it hard for them to accuse me of being lazy or lacking in motivation. On the contrary, they might even think that my problem had been caused by working too hard and doing too much training. It was almost as if it were a 'respectable' way of getting CFS. Also, the life of a sportsman is often seen as glamorous, not something that one would want to withdraw from voluntarily. Quite unfairly, these factors perhaps gave me more credibility than other sufferers. I sympathised with them. Many people had developed the illness while holding down more conventional jobs. Like me, they found it hard to get treatment and even harder to explain their illness. They had a difficult time trying to convince their employers and workmates that they needed to take a year off work.

I was fortunate because most people were very supportive and genuinely concerned about me. This sometimes became a bit boring for fellow players and close friends like Simon Parke and Alex Gough, who became unofficial spokesmen to the world of squash about the state of my health. They complained that wherever they went in the world to play a tournament, they were constantly being asked how I was by fans and other players. Alex said he'd even considered recording his answer so he could hand people a tape whenever they asked!

From the time I first started feeling unwell in the summer of 1994, I had become very focused on my illness and the anguish it was causing. However, in December 1996 something happened that made me forget all about my problems and turn my attention to something far more serious. Simon Parke discovered he was suffering from testicular cancer. The news sent a shock wave through his friends and family as well as squash fans everywhere. Testicular cancer is the biggest cause of cancer deaths in young men under 30. Simon was hit very badly, and had to undergo chemotherapy. He lost all his hair and was told that although there was a 95 per cent chance that he would recover, he might not have the strength to play professional squash again. It was obviously a traumatic time for him but he's always been a tremendously determined character. Thankfully, he caught it early enough and responded well to treatment. He was out of the game for six months, and although his life was no longer in danger, it was by no means certain that he would be able to go back to playing squash. For a while it looked as though both our careers might be over.

There was more bad news to come. Another friend from childhood, David Campion, got a bad back injury and had to stop playing. He had similar experiences to me, going to see various doctors. None of them seemed to know what was wrong or how he was going to put it right. People were telling him to try all sorts of different treatments like ultrasound and massage, but none of them worked. Like me, he was getting frustrated and started to lose hope. It was strange how all three of us had problems at the same time given that we were so young. We had come into the game together and now it seemed we were going out together. We met up a few times during this period to talk about it and try to cheer ourselves up. Despite the seriousness of the situation, we were able to laugh about it. We had started as youngsters dreaming of beating the world, and here we were like a bunch of old crocks before we had barely started. Where did it all go wrong? Simon joked that it was probably all my fault – I had been ill for so long that I had put a jinx on them.

Although we were out of the game, many of our contractual obligations continued. In 1996, Simon and I had to attend the British National Championships because it was part of our deal with our sponsors. That was very hard. We had to watch other players competing for the trophy we thought we should be out there winning. We had to experience the atmosphere of the big occasion knowing that for the first time we weren't really part of it. In the back of our minds, we feared we might never be part of it again. It was like rubbing salt in our wounds.

Peter Nicol beat Mark Chaloner in the final. It was a great game between two very good players, but we weren't interested. The fans and everyone connected with the game were very supportive. Lots of people came up to talk to us and ask about our health. They meant well, and we appreciated their concern, but we didn't really want to be there talking about it. I don't want to wish any ill on Simon, but I was glad in a way that he was there with me because it made it a bit easier.

Thankfully, Simon made a full recovery from his illness and was able to make a successful return to the circuit. I remember thinking there was a big change in him when he started playing again. He seemed less pressured. When he found out that he could still play at the top level, it was obviously a tremendous relief. He seemed to regard everything as a bonus and was determined just to enjoy his life and his squash as much as possible. I told myself that if I ever managed to start playing again, I would remember how he had handled his return. I would try to have the same attitude and enjoy it as much as possible. It's easy to see your career as being all-important. That attitude soon changes when your health and life are threatened.

# 7.

## FOR LOVE OR MONEY

People thought I was mad. I was out of work with no immediate prospects of making a living, yet I was turning down a quarter of a million pounds. All I had to do was sign on the dotted line and walk away a rich young man. It was mine for the taking, but I was rejecting it without a moment's hesitation. It wasn't that I didn't appreciate the money. It was a very generous offer. The problem was that it had a huge drawback; it would have meant never playing professional squash again. To some people that might have been a small price to pay, but to me it was unthinkable. I wasn't interested in the money. I was desperate to get back on court.

The offer came about because I was insured in the event of injury or illness ending my career prematurely and depriving me of my livelihood. The policy provided me with a monthly allowance when my income from squash dried up. It also entitled me to take a quarter of a million pounds as a lump sum if it turned out my career was truly over. I had been out of the game for nearly two years with little prospect of returning, and so my insurance company was willing to pay me off. Obviously, if I accepted their settlement I couldn't have started playing again at a later date, or they could have sued me. The money would have set me up for life. It wasn't as if there was much prospect of me setting the world of squash alight at that point. Very few people come back after a two-year absence and compete at the top level. Not only that, but I wasn't really over my illness yet. No definite cure had been found and although I was feeling better, I still wasn't 100 per cent right. If I did decide to make a comeback, there was no guarantee that my health wouldn't break down again.

This is where the insurance policy provided the cruellest twist of all. If I spurned the pay-off and returned to the professional circuit, even if it was only for one game before my health gave way again, I would lose all my rights to any insurance money in the future. This was because the policy would only pay out once for any particular illness. I had already made my claim for CFS and would not be able to make another, no matter how ill I became, if I made an abortive comeback attempt. There was no way to hedge my bets. It was all or nothing: either go with the money and give up the game, or go with the game and give up the money.

A lot of people thought it would be better to take the insurance company's offer, but to me it was never an issue. I enjoyed being a squash player. It was what I knew and it was what I enjoyed doing. I still felt very frustrated at having to withdraw from the game after working so hard to reach the world number two slot. I was convinced I could have gone on to be number one if my health hadn't failed. There was still a large part of me that wanted to claim that number one position. I wanted to prove that I could do it, to myself as much as anyone else.

I also wanted to get back on the circuit. Like most players, I suppose I had taken it all for granted while I had been playing. It was only when it was taken away from me that I realised what a great lifestyle it was. Anyone who complains about it isn't living in the real world. Players treat it differently, of course. For some, it's just a passport to travel around the world enjoying themselves while they're young and carefree. Others take it more seriously and are focused on winning tournaments.

The lifestyle suited me perfectly. You have to train hard, obviously, but then you're free to do whatever you want with your time. I don't think I ever woke up one morning thinking that I didn't want to do it any more, or that I was fed up of the training. It always brought something different. One day you might be competing in a major tournament, staying at one of the best hotels in the world; the next you might be sleeping on someone's floor after playing some minor league match. It was unpredictable and it suited me.

Martin Heath describes me as something of a free spirit; someone who doesn't conform to the usual conventions but prefers to tread his own path. It may sometimes be a lonely path; it may even be the wrong path. But the point is that it's entirely my own. Being a squash player enabled me to be myself in a way that would be hard to achieve in any other profession. I was my own boss, answerable to no one but myself. I was my main source of motivation and also my own main critic. I stood or fell on my own, and I liked that. At the other extreme I liked and missed the company of the other players. The Park club in Nottingham has become a hotbed for professional squash over the last few years. Simon Parke, Alex Gough, Derek Ryan and John White all live in the city and train there, and the England team often meet at the club, bringing more top players like Paul Johnson, Del Harris and Chris Walker. I was seeing them all regularly while I was ill, but it wasn't the same as being able to train with them and compete against them. I just didn't feel part of it all. That was hard, because I had known many of those people for most of my life.

I particularly missed my battles with Simon. We had played each other in numerous tournaments around the world, but I sometimes think the public have never seen our most fiercely fought encounters. These were the ordinary practice matches back home in Nottingham with nobody watching except perhaps a bored cleaner or barman. We could compete for thousands of pounds in important tournaments and not think too much about it, but what really brought out our competitive instinct was who would buy the drinks after training. As soon as it was agreed the loser had to pay, we would both pull out all the stops. A routine training match could last two hours and go to five games. People who had seen us both behaving impeccably in tournaments might well be shocked to see us falling out and arguing over disputed points and let calls. After all, there was beer at stake! Eventually, we would stagger off court drained and drenched in sweat. Joy for the winner; humiliation for the loser. And then, of course, to the victor the spoils. I don't think either of us ever enjoyed a drink so much as when we forced the other one to pay for it. I never realised how much I enjoyed silly moments like that until they were taken away from me. I also missed the camaraderie with the other players as we travelled together to the world's top tournaments.

Players are very competitive on court, but tend to get on quite well once the match is over. Often we would all be staying in the same hotels, and there was always a lot of socialising. Players had to be very careful while they were in the tournament, but as soon as they were knocked out they would be looking to relax and enjoy themselves. As the tournament went on, more players would of course get knocked out, and so the party would get bigger. I remembered having some great nights on the circuit and it pained me to no longer be part of it.

I also missed the contact with the fans. Because squash is still a relatively minor sport, the tournaments tend to be quite open and relaxed. Players don't have vast sums of money thrown at them so they don't develop prima donna tendencies as they do in some more lucrative sports. Everyone is down to earth and friendly. Players will often mingle with the crowds when they're not competing, and this makes them very accessible to the fans. I had enjoyed all that and missed it as I sat at home in Nottingham.

The thing I missed the most, though, was the thrill of competing. Before my illness, I was like most other pros and might feel glad to see the end of the season approach so I could relax and take a holiday. But within a month or two, I would be getting restless and itching for the new season to start. After two years out of the game, I felt that way ten times over. It's hard to describe the buzz of competing and the thrill of winning. There's nothing quite like it. The game drives you to extremes. You're ecstatic when you win; you're distraught when you lose. There's nothing in between. Thankfully, the joy of the victories tends to outweigh the pain of the defeats. After losing, you might feel down for an hour or two but you soon snap out of it. You can always go and unwind with some of the other unfortunates who've lost out. And, of course, there's always another tournament around the corner to give you the chance to put things right.

All of those factors were gnawing away at me, making me want to return to the game. What they illustrate, I suppose, is my love of playing squash. Martin Heath has a theory that when people get involved in professional sport they start to play it down. They hide their enthusiasm for the game – they want to be like everyone else. I never thought that way at all. I'll talk all day about squash to anyone, and that is one of the things Martin latched on to immediately when we first met. He was struck by the fact that I was totally comfortable with my interest in the game. Martin is passionate about squash, and says my unashamed enthusiasm gave him confidence that it was all right. As he says, spending hours hitting a ball down the side of a wall, not just because it's your job, not even because you enjoy it but because you have a real passion for the game, might seem a little odd to the outside world. He likens it to the obsessions some people might have about climbing Everest or swimming the channel. They're small passions, they're not particularly significant, but they're real. People who follow them have confidence in what they're doing even though it may appear odd to others.

Whatever the case, like Martin, I was smitten with the game and everything surrounding it. It's hardly surprising, then, that I wanted to get back to playing as quickly as possible. The only question mark in my mind was the state of my health. By October 1996, I had been out of the game for a year and a half. I had followed Dr Budgett's advice and got plenty of rest. It paid off to a certain extent. I gradually started to feel stronger. The sore throats were becoming less frequent and I was sleeping a lot better. As I improved physically, I could feel myself changing mentally. My drive was coming back. When you're ill, your body won't let you perform. This can make you feel that you're no longer keen to play, but really it's just that you don't have the energy. Once that energy starts to return, your spirit perks up. That's what happened to me.

I built up my training gradually. I found that my muscles weren't getting as tired or filling with lactic acid so quickly. It was possible to work quite hard without feeling exhausted the next day. This gave me a boost and I started going back on court to practise by myself. Thankfully, I didn't feel too bad. I also played the occasional game against players who weren't going to push me very hard. My positive feelings started to come back and I wanted to get back on a squash court and play competitively. It was a time of increasing hope. I felt much better – but had I made enough improvement? Despite my progress, I still wasn't fully recovered. There was a lot to think about. A year and a half is a long time relaxing and it's certainly a long time out of a squash career. Maybe rest and a gentle approach to training had done all they could for me, and I had reached a plateau. Maybe the thing to do was to go for it 100 per cent and build up my training to the level it had been before I became ill.

I spoke to the doctors about this and they didn't object, although they advised caution. They suggested I play a few more practice matches against players who were considerably below my standard just to get me back into it. I tried this, and it seemed to work okay. Then I played Simon Parke and he was so much better than me that it would have been embarrassing if he weren't such a good friend. I knew he was going easy on me, too, which made it worse. Playing Simon made me realise how far I had fallen behind. Still, it was good to be on court and I felt better just for that.

I went to see Dr Scott again. This time she advised me to try a drug called Phenelzine, another anti-depressant, but also a kind of energiser. She said it had helped other sufferers. The theory was that if you've been ill for a long time, you can start to feel down mentally. If you can take something to make you feel better mentally, it might get the ball rolling to help you get stronger physically as well. I took the Phenelzine, and I did notice an improvement. I wasn't sure if it was down to the drug or whether I was at last feeling the benefit of the rest I'd been taking. I think I also got a boost from being back on court. Whatever the reason, I felt strong enough to try a more competitive match again just to see how I would get on, so I played Adam Toes in the Yorkshire league. He was ranked about 25 in England and I beat him 3–1. Normally I wouldn't have expected to lose a game against him, but under the circumstances I was delighted. I increased my training, doing two hard sessions a week interspersed with low and medium intensity programmes.

I continued to make progress, and in January 1997 I went back to see Dr Scott. She increased the dose of Phenelzine. I was now feeling much more positive. I continued playing, including several more practice matches against Simon, and was very pleased with my progress. I still wasn't anywhere near as strong as I used to be and although my symptoms were better, I still wasn't sure that I was cured. Nevertheless, I felt confident enough to try a comeback.

It was good to make such a positive decision. That was a boost in itself. I was still far from 100 per cent but hoped that things would get better as I went along. My training was going well and I was reasonably confident. Until the Phenelzine started creating some worrying side effects. I started to suffer from anxiety and found it hard to rest. Sometimes I was only sleeping for about two hours. My body felt full of adrenaline. I was tired, yet felt alert. I got dizzy sometimes when I was playing. I wasn't sure what to do. Part of me wanted to stop taking the drugs, but another part of me thought it would be better to persevere. Then it got to the point where I could only sleep for about an hour a night. There was no relaxation, because the Phenelzine was a form of stimulant. I felt high all the time, as if I was wired up. I started to lose my appetite. Then the dizziness worsened, to the point where I couldn't play at all.

It was very worrying and I felt as though I was being driven to mental exhaustion. It was March by now, and only a few weeks away from the game's biggest tournament, the British Open. I desperately wanted to play in it. I needed to feel better, not only for my health's sake, but to be fit enough to compete. I persevered with the Phenelzine for about two months but decided it was counter-productive. Three weeks before the start of the British Open in March I decided to stop taking it. I had hoped for an immediate improvement, but things got worse. I started to get withdrawal symptoms. My body wanted the drug and I started to feel even more anxious than when I was taking it. I was feeling down and almost paranoid. It was a horrible time. I was adamant at that time that I wouldn't take any more drugs, of any kind.

Thankfully, the withdrawal symptoms only lasted a few weeks and by the start of the tournament, I was returning to normal. Although, at this point, 'normal' was nowhere near as good as I felt before I became ill. In the first round I was drawn against Brett Martin, the player I had beaten in the semi-final two years before in a match that had left me exhausted and made me finally realise that something serious was wrong. I was looking forward to the game but not really expecting too much, and so it turned out. I managed to stay with him to 12–12 in the first game, but that was it. He was a tough opponent at the best of times, but I lacked fitness and match practice and he beat me quite easily in three games. I wasn't too disappointed. I was just pleased to be there. I was coming to believe that I would never recover fully, so just being able to play at all was a bonus.

I felt very tired after the British Open and needed to rest for about a week before I felt as well as before the tournament started. I didn't mind too much at that point, because it had been my first major event for two years. I decided that the next tournament I would play would be the Al Ahram in Egypt, in May. That gave me six weeks to prepare. I built up my training programme in the hope of getting somewhere near the level I was at before I became ill. I was managing to cope, but was disappointed that it wasn't getting any easier.

I lost to the local hero, Ahmed Barada. He was developing into a major force on the circuit and it was no shame to lose to him, but it showed me that I was still a long way from being fully fit. It was frustrating but I consoled myself with the thought that the season was over and I now had the summer to prepare properly for the following year.

I trained hard over the next few months. Then, in August, I set off for the first big tournament of the new season, the Hong Kong Open. I was fitter now than at any point since my withdrawal, so this would be a good test of how far I had come. In the first round, I beat Anthony Hill who was in the world top ten. Then I beat the world number two, Rodney Eyles. That game carried a huge significance for me because it showed I could still compete at the very top level despite being out for so long. The euphoria was short-lived, however, and I lost to Brett Martin the following day. He was still a good way ahead of me but at least I got much closer to him than I had in the British Open.

All that was very positive, but there were worrying developments when I got home. I felt totally drained and it took me a long time to recover. It was nearly two weeks before I could start training again. Even then, I felt exhausted. I told myself that perhaps it was just that I had been out of the game for two years, and it would obviously take a long time to get back to normal. Deep down, though, I didn't really believe that. I wasn't sure what to do. I was worried about what I was doing to my body by putting it through so much when it clearly was struggling to cope. If I was going to feel like this after every tournament, I wouldn't be able to continue. I decided to think positively and press on. Perhaps everything would come right once I got more tournaments behind me.

The US Open came just three weeks after Hong Kong, so by the time I had recovered there was no time to do any training. I just had to fly out there. I played Ahmed Barada, who had beaten me in Egypt. This time I won 3–0 and followed it up with another win over Rodney Eyles before going out 3–2 to Simon Parke. Everyone was very positive and told me I was doing brilliantly considering I had been out of the game for so long. Part of me agreed, but I also felt frustrated. Before I became ill I had been used to getting to the final of most competitions, and now I always seemed to be going out in the early rounds. Maybe I was expecting too much, but I couldn't help feeling that I ought to be doing better.

I felt even worse after the US Open than I had after Hong Kong. Far from getting stronger as I played more tournaments, I seemed to be getting weaker. I had struggled physically during most of the matches and it took a big mental effort to get through them. As I rested back home in England, I was paying the price. I was exhausted and it wasn't the normal kind of tiredness that comes after a lot of exertion. I could tell that I still had CFS, although I didn't like having to admit it to myself.

The only question was what to do about it. I wondered if I should withdraw again and rest until I felt better. The problem was that I had already rested for a year and a half and had little to show for it. I had improved, of course, but I still couldn't play at my full capacity and I was taking too long to recover. I thought of those doctors who argued that the best thing was to ignore the problem and just carry on as normal. Perhaps it was largely psychological, and I should just get on with it. I had already entered for the World Open in Malaysia. Should I pull out, or give it another go and see what happened?

I agonised over it for days, but in the end I decided to go for it. As far as my health was concerned, what difference would one tournament make? I could always rest afterwards. I set off and hoped for the best. It was about three weeks since the US Open and I had spent most of that time resting. I was in no fit state to train. For the third time that year, I came up against Brett Martin. This time I beat him, although it was another marathon effort that went to five games. Afterwards, journalists put the victory down to the twin pillars of my game, my powers of endurance and indomitable spirit. I certainly needed every ounce of those qualities to get through, because I was definitely feeling the pace. Thankfully, I got through the next round against Dan Jensen a little easier. Then, in the next round, I came up against the player who more than anyone else had been setting the game alight while I had been out.

Jonathan Power had been winning tournaments with what often seemed like effortless performances. Apart from Jansher Khan, he was probably playing better than anyone else at that time and was soon to become the world number one. With Jansher out of the tournament suffering from tonsillitis, Power was the favourite to win and become world champion. The game created a lot of interest among fans because I was coming back from an illness, and they wanted to see how I would perform against the rising star. I was looking forward to it as well. It was a great chance to see how far I had progressed. I knew I wasn't at my best, but I desperately wanted to win.

I took the first game, but it was very close at 15–12. The second was even closer, 15–14. That took a lot out of me, and the third was a nightmare. I was struggling to find any energy and folded completely, losing 15–2. At least it gave me a breather and I came out for the fourth determined to regain the initiative. It worked better than I could have hoped, and I raced ahead to a 13–4 lead. I thought I had him but, showing an indomitable spirit of his own, he fought his way back, playing a series of the fantastically deceptive winning shots that had become his trademark. Suddenly it was 13–9 and he was on a roll. His step was quickening, as if he could sense that he might yet pull it back. He would have known that I was likely to tire if he could keep me in the game long enough. I tried to hold myself together and decided to step up the pace for one last effort to get back in front. Power fought me all the way, but he didn't get another point. I won 15–9. I was delighted. I had beaten the hottest player on the circuit and felt that at last I was back. My joy was short lived, unfortunately. Once the adrenaline and excitement wore off, I felt totally drained.

That game against Power was similar in effect to the British Open semi-final against Brett Martin two years earlier. I won, but it took too much out of me. I spoke to Jonah Barrington about it afterwards and he said it seemed as though I had played to a higher level than my body was capable of maintaining. My ability and experience meant I was able to compete with Power on equal terms, but I lacked the physical strength. I had made up for that on the day through determination and willpower. I was motivated by the emotion of wanting to play again after being out for so long. There was the drama of the occasion, the quarter-final of the world open. It all acted like a stimulant to me and I was able to summon everything I had to pull myself through. It was the kind of thing I could only do once, unfortunately, because I was at the limits of my body's capability. Considering the state of my health, it was one of the best performances of my life, but there was no way I could push myself like that on a regular basis. I knew that if I was to play Power another five times that month he would have beaten me every time.

My opponent in the semi-final was Rodney Eyles, whom I had already beaten twice since my comeback. I won the opening game but then couldn't summon up enough energy to compete. Eyles took it easily. I don't want to take anything away from him, because he was playing some of the best squash of his career. He went on to beat Peter Nicol in the final so there was no denying he was in great form – I might not have beaten him no matter how fit I had been – but I was disappointed that I hadn't been able to compete properly.

A week later, I headed off to Bombay to compete in the Mahindra International Challenge. In the first round, I came up against Peter Nicol. He was seeded second behind Jansher Khan who had returned after his illness. The last time I had played Nicol was three years earlier, when I had beaten him in the semi-final of the World Open in Barcelona. This time the tables were turned. I managed to get a game but he won relatively easily. I just wasn't able to put up any resistance.

It was time to take stock. I had performed well in the World Open and had a good tournament, but I didn't feel I could carry on that way. I was barely able to recover from one event before it was time to go and compete in another. Other players were fitting in league matches, exhibition games and minor tournaments in between those big occasions but all I was able to do was rest. I went back home feeling very despondent. My long lay-off had obviously done me a lot of good, but I still wasn't able to play professional squash in the way that I wanted. I was as good as anyone in individual matches but I didn't have the energy to sustain a whole tournament. On that basis, I was never going to win anything and I ran the risk of doing serious damage to my health in the attempt.

I rested over Christmas in the hope of recharging my batteries, but my recovery was very slow. I caught flu which obviously didn't help. I wasn't feeling much better as I went into the New Year and pulled out of the British National Championships, which was a big disappointment to me as it was a tournament I had always enjoyed. While I should have been thinking about preparing for the British Open which was coming up, I just didn't have the energy. I struggled on into February and March playing a few league matches and trying to find a way forward, but it was no use. I felt continually exhausted, the CFS was back as bad as ever. There seemed to be nothing I could do. I reconciled myself to another long lay-off and had no idea whether I would ever be able to come back.

# 8.

# A LIFE MORE ORDINARY

My failed comeback attempt left me even worse off than before. My illness was as bad as ever, but now I had far less confidence that I could recover. I no longer believed that the medical profession could help me. After my second breakdown, I went to see my GP and the only thing he could advise me to do was rest. I thought, 'What's the point in that? I've already tried that and it did no good.' He had nothing else to offer. At least he was being honest. That was more than could be said for some of the people who had treated me in the past. I had travelled all over the world, to the United States and throughout Europe, speaking to so-called experts on the subject. None of them could provide an answer.

If I had learnt anything during my illness, it was that the medical profession doesn't fully understand CFS. That isn't their fault: not enough research has been done on it. Most doctors acknowledged this and said things like: 'No one can find a single cure but this medication has been known to help some people so why not try it?' I could accept that approach. People like Dr Budgett, Dr Scott and Mike Ash were professional and very straight with me. They made no false promises, and they gave me some good advice.

Sadly, there were some people, mainly those who specialised in alternative remedies, who had very fixed ideas and acted as if they knew exactly what to do. Some of them only seemed to be in it for the money. They would say things like: 'It's definitely such-and-such a problem and if you take this, this and this you'll be fine.' I remember looking at such people and thinking: 'Well, what do you know really? This is a complex issue, yet you think you have the answer and you make it sound so simple. I don't believe you. It can't be that easy.' Many of these alternative therapists seemed convinced that their approach was the best and the only one that would work. They would often rubbish mainstream medicine and even other therapists. I quickly concluded that the more convinced they were that they were right, the more likely they were to be wrong. I much preferred the open-minded approach of the doctors who provided most of my care.

No matter how much I felt I could see through these self-styled experts, however, I was still drawn to them. I was desperate for a cure. Some of the alternative therapists I had encountered were conscientious and professional, but all too often they would glibly dole out advice and then sting me with a £500 bill for something that did no good at all. That's a lot of money when you're not earning. Even more damaging was the frustration of having my hopes built up only to have them come crashing down again.

One set of therapists I saw specialised in nutrition and herbal remedies to provide extra energy. They were convinced that I would quickly recover if I took the tablets they gave me, together with vitamin supplements and various nutrients extracted from herbal components. I went to see them a couple of times and ended up paying them more than £700. Their wonder supplements did me no good at all. I wasn't particularly surprised and neither, I think, were they. I felt they were preying on people's desperation to get better.

As I looked back, I realised I had probably been naive to listen to such people. Perhaps I shouldn't be too critical, because they can always claim that their methods worked for others. All I can say was that they didn't work for me. I didn't want to go through it all again the second time around. I resolved to stop searching for treatments and just let nature take its course. I might start to feel better, but if I didn't I would be no worse off than when I had been wasting my time with so-called experts who had nothing to offer.

I began to take stock. I hoped to return to the game, but had to accept that that was now even more unlikely. In the meantime, I would have to find new ways of making a living. I was no longer entitled to any insurance money. Perhaps the people who thought I was mad not to take the quarter of a million pounds pay-off were right, but I never saw it that way. I was glad I had taken a chance on rebuilding my career. If I hadn't, I would have regretted it for the rest of my life and forever wondered about what might have been. At least I would never be tortured by that kind of uncertainty.

For a while I thought that I might take up coaching. I felt I had a lot of valuable experience to offer younger players. I went to a few of the national training squads for talented youngsters and started helping out. Normally, I would have really enjoyed it but under the circumstances, I found it a hard concept to deal with. It was very difficult to be around squash players when I couldn't play myself, and going along seemed to be emphasising my plight rather than taking my mind off it. I went a few times but then gave it up. I thought I would be better off trying to do something totally different, outside the game.

Journalism seemed appealing, but I realised I would have to get more academic qualifications. I had all my GCSEs but they wouldn't be enough. During my previous lay-off, I had done courses in biology and sports science. Now I wanted a fresh challenge so I chose A Level English. I was studying a range of authors, from Shakespeare to the black American writer Maya Angelou. It was very stimulating and I could lose myself in it. There were times when I felt very positive. I realised there were some advantages to being out of the game. My thinking became much broader and more varied. When you're playing, everything revolves around squash. It's not just the four or five hours a day training; it's everything that goes with that. It fills your mind all the time and constantly influences how you live your life. You might not be able to go out with friends because you have to rest for a match the next day or you have to eat at a certain time. You can't let your hair down because you have to train the following morning. You miss out on time with family and friends because you're forever away at tournaments. I had been doing that since I was a teenager, and now that I was out of the game, I realised how abnormal it was to live that way. Part of me enjoyed the prospect of a more ordinary life with fewer disruptions and restrictions on what I could do.

I rested for the first few months of 1998, and although there was some improvement in my condition there was still a long way to go. I still felt tired and lethargic, and my mood could be very low. It was hard to know what to do about it. I was desperate to feel better. Not so much so that I could play squash, but just for the sake of my general health and my future. If I were to make the most of a new life and a new career, I would have to regain my full strength. I found myself tempted again by a variety of different therapies. I subscribed to various newsletters about CFS and these often carried articles about treatments people had found useful. A lot of people, including friends, fellow sufferers and squash fans, had also written to me suggesting new ideas. I began to look seriously at these, even though some of them appeared a little bizarre: things like reflexology, magnetism, osteopathy, magnesium injection, acupuncture and so on. Deep down I knew that they were unlikely to work because most of them had only a limited scientific basis. I was also determined not to allow myself to be exploited again. Nevertheless, I would say to myself: 'Yes, it does sound unlikely, but what alternative do you have? What if it turns out that this is the thing that could finally cure you? Other people say it's worked for them. You have to try it, if only to put your mind at rest. Otherwise you could regret it later.'

That was how I found myself walking around with a magnet strapped to my wrist. I even had to wear it in bed. The theory was that CFS sufferers might have some disruption to their magnetic field and this could weaken their energy source. Wearing the magnet was supposed to correct this imbalance. As far as I'm aware people don't actually have their own magnetic fields, but in my desperation I was prepared to overlook this. I wore the magnets for three or four days. As I suspected all along, they did no good. I took them off, feeling a little sheepish and perhaps even angry with myself for trying such long shots. At least I couldn't complain about the honesty of the therapists, as they had made no false claims. I was careful to avoid people who were too full of themselves and thought they had an answer for everything.

I had some tests done that suggested my condition might have been caused by a lack of magnesium, which the body needs to enable the muscles to create energy effectively. If I had a deficiency it might explain my muscle fatigue. I started taking magnesium sulphate tablets and I also had to have injections. These were directly into the muscle in the leg and were extremely painful. I endured this for six weeks but then gave it up. They were making no difference at all. This was particularly disappointing, as I had really thought it might work. Later I discovered that magnesium injection was highly controversial, with many doctors sceptical about its value. I wish I had known that before I agreed to endure the pain of the injections.

Acupuncture was once scoffed at by western doctors but is now taken more seriously. The Chinese believe that energy flows through the body along channels to and from the vital organs such as the heart and lungs. It is thought that if there's a disease in one of those organs it can disrupt the flow of energy. The job of the acupuncturist is to decide where the problem is and then insert needles into the body to correct any malfunctioning. The difficulty with this theory from a western point of view is that the energy channels don't correspond to any known system within the body. You can't see them, or detect them in any way. On the other hand, for whatever reason, acupuncture works for a lot of people so it can't be easily dismissed. It can sometimes relieve suffering where conventional painkillers fail and can even be used as an anaesthetic. Many pregnant women have found it useful during labour.

I still wasn't really sold on the idea, but I thought that perhaps I should try it. No one was claiming it could cure CFS, but many people believed that it had helped to relieve their symptoms. This may be because acupuncture encourages the body to release endorphins, which act as painkillers. I read this thinking that maybe this was the approach I should take. Perhaps it was time to lower my sights, stop looking for a cure and settle for a way simply to reduce the symptoms. I tried it, and found it was far less painful than I had feared. That was the only positive thing, unfortunately. It didn't work for me at all. My condition remained the same.

It was now the summer of 1998 and I was showing few signs of improvement. At least my studies were going well. I was reading the story of Maya Angelou and how she overcame the abuse, discrimination and poverty that came with being a black woman in the American south of the 1930s. Getting inside the traumas faced by someone else helped me to forget my own problems, if only for a while. I was also grappling with Shakespeare's *Hamlet* and *King Lear*, Ian McEwan's *The Cement Garden* and *Uncle Tom's Cabin* by Harriet Beecher-Stowe. They all took me into worlds far removed from the squash court.

There was no lasting escape, however, and my lost career was always coming back into my mind. I was often filled with a sense of what might have been. By this time, Jansher Khan was starting to fade and if it hadn't been for my health, I would have been his natural successor. Instead, the baton was being passed to the next generation of top players, led by Peter Nicol and Jonathan Power. They were now sharing the number one and two spots. It seemed ironic. I had beaten Peter Nicol 3–0 to win the British National Championship in 1994. I had beaten Power 3–1 during my comeback in the quarter-final of the World Open, even though I wasn't fully match fit. I was sure I could beat them again if only I could regain my health. That possibility seemed a long way off, however, and I knew I had to put such thoughts out of my mind as they were getting me nowhere.

I wondered what to do next and found myself trying more alternative treatments. The CFS newsletters contained many reports of people who had found reflexology useful. It works on the assumption that practitioners can detect the cause of illnesses by examining the soles of the feet. Once the diagnosis has been made, the idea is to massage the foot and toes in a particular way to clear blocked energy channels and restore health. It didn't sound very probable, but I had nothing to lose, so I tried it. The reflexologist didn't say she could cure me, but she said the treatment could help me feel better. It was very relaxing and I could see how it might benefit people suffering from some illnesses, particularly those that are stress-related, but it didn't do anything for me. It was back to square one.

After flirting with so many fringe treatments, I wanted something that was a little more mainstream, if not completely conventional. I turned to osteopathy, a treatment mainly concerned with treating back pain but used more and more by people suffering from CFS. I was encouraged to see that a trial group of CFS patients had shown significant improvement after receiving treatment. When I went to see an osteopath he suggested that the problem was linked to the nervous system in my back. He gave me a series of stretching exercises to increase the flexibility of the spine. These were quite difficult, and took a lot of dedication. I had to do them six times a day. There were also some co-ordination exercises that took another 40 minutes a day, so it was quite an extensive programme. Another part of the treatment was to place ice packs on the spine. This was supposed to increase the blood supply to the area and so speed up the healing process. On top of this, I had to have massages as well, to get rid of the toxic waste that CFS produces.

I stuck to it rigidly but after a while I started to lose confidence. I didn't feel it was doing me any good. I was confused. Part of me thought that I had to keep going no matter what, and the other part told me I should stop because it wasn't going to work. The lack of benefit seemed out of all proportion to the effort involved, and I found myself feeling angry and hostile about the whole thing. I felt I would rather do nothing than waste time on something that didn't work. I gave up after about four months.

It was now October, and I was feeling really down because nothing I tried seemed to make me feel any better. Then, just when I thought I couldn't feel much worse, I switched on satellite television and saw something that brought me down even further. Peter Nicol and Jonathan Power were slugging it out in one of their many gripping matches. This was a little different, however. They weren't just playing for themselves. They were playing for their countries in the final of the Commonwealth Games: Scotland against Canada. I had played in all the major tournaments several times, but never in anything like the Commonwealth Games.

To my surprise, I found it very hard to take and felt that sick, panicky sensation in the stomach that you get when something frightens or alarms you. More than ever, I felt I was really missing out. Deep down, I desperately wanted to be out there on court competing with Power and Nicol. It wasn't so much that I thought I could beat them, although I would have fancied my chances – it was just that I wanted to be there. It sickened me to think I would never be a part of it. This was a surprisingly extreme reaction, but then I was probably at my lowest ebb at the time.

One of my biggest regrets at being out was that it prevented me playing Jansher Khan several more times and hopefully beating him. Any professional wants to test himself against the best, and Jansher certainly came into that category. I will always wonder whether I would have gone on to overtake him at the top if I had not become ill. Jonah Barrington said he thought that Jansher eased off a little after I stopped playing because there was no one else who could push him. He lost a little fitness because he didn't have to work as hard and was fading at that time as he was getting older. I think I would have succeeded him as the world number one had I been able to keep playing. Knowing that was very frustrating.

As it turned out, it was left to others to take up the challenge. Jansher was getting more and more out of condition and many younger players tried to exploit this by keeping him on court as long as possible in order to tire him, hoping that if they could drain him mentally and physically he would eventually lose heart or simply run out of energy. Peter Nicol was the first player to do this successfully, and he eventually beat Jansher in the Egyptian Open in '97. Jansher battled on for another year or so, but his air of invulnerability had gone and he eventually retired from the scene. I was sad to see him go. It was the end of an era, an era in which I had played a significant part. I felt I had been robbed of the opportunity to fulfil my potential by taking over from him.

The following few months were a very bad time for me. There seemed no escape from my illness and I had to do a lot of soul-searching about what I was doing, where I was going and whether any of it was worthwhile. None of the treatments I had tried had any beneficial effect. Not only that, but my desperation was making me try ever more fanciful treatments. Sometimes when I looked back on them or discussed them with others I would feel stupid. I could see they thought it was ridiculous to expect that wearing magnets or having foot massages could cure a debilitating illness. I thought it was ridiculous too, but was driven on by an ever more desperate search for something that could help. It was damaging to my self-esteem. I may have been ill, but I deserved better than to clutch at treatments that had no prospect of being successful.

It was typical of me to tell myself that I should try a cure, no matter how bizarre, because it could just be the one that works. It wasn't in my nature to give in. I had spent all my life battling to win, to succeed, and to overcome every obstacle to achieve my ambition to get to the top in squash. It was hardly surprising that I should apply the same determination to beat my illness. In the end, however, I felt that the search itself was becoming part of the problem. For four years, I had been building up my hopes with each new treatment only to come crashing down again when they failed to work. It was becoming counter-productive. The constant disappointment was making me feel worse. It's good to be a fighter and have a never-say-die attitude. But there are limits, even for someone described by the *Guardian* newspaper as 'the most stubborn man in the history of squash'. There was no point in torturing myself any more. There had to come a point when I accepted that enough was enough.

All that was easy enough to say, but was it really the way forward? Could I cope with never playing again? Was this really the end of my career? Surely I wasn't really going to give in? It was contrary to my nature. Wouldn't the frustration of giving up be even worse than the frustration of searching fruitlessly for a cure? I wasn't sure. I found myself in the conundrum faced by many people who have to make a major change in lifestyle, whether it's trying to stop smoking, lose weight, cut down on drinking, whatever. It's easy to recognise what you have to do; the hard part is actually doing it. I had to come to terms with the fact that I would probably never find a cure or play at the top level again. I understood this but then, just as I thought I had come to terms with it all, I would relapse into anger and frustration, as I had done watching Nicol and Power at the Commonwealth Games.

At this point I started to wonder if my psychological state was becoming part of the problem. Throughout my illness, I had always tried to remain positive and maintain the traditional British stiff upper lip. I didn't want to feel sorry for myself or go around berating the world, saying 'Why me?' But, in reality, it was hard not to feel down. The stress and anxiety I was feeling in my desperate search for a cure were taking their toll. Perhaps there was a danger that I had got into a vicious circle. It was possible that after a while my mental state had stopped being the effect of my illness and had started becoming the cause, at least in part. Perhaps I had got into a mental rut and needed a kick-start to get me thinking positively again. Maybe that would improve my physical condition.

I tried to look at my personality to see if there was something there that could be contributing to the illness. Perhaps my energies had been channelled too much in one direction. According to the experts, certain characters were more prone than others to suffer from things like CFS: people who were highly ambitious were particularly at risk; sometimes they allow their careers to assume too much importance. They won't let anything to stand in the way of what they want to achieve. Consequently, if they become ill they may be so frightened of losing ground that they return to work too soon. They don't allow themselves enough time to recover. Instead, they work harder and harder to get on the next rung of the ladder, and after a while they forget why they're doing it. This is counter-productive – before they know it, all the other areas of their lives such as their health and relationships begin to suffer, even though those other areas may be more important in the long run.

I looked at my childhood. I remembered all those early matches I played when I became the British Under-10 champion and then followed it up with the Under-12 title in the same year, even though I was two years younger than the other boys. How was I able to overcome the age gap and beat them? Was I simply a more talented player? Or was it that I wanted it more than they did? I didn't know, but I remembered how incredibly important squash was to me, even at that early age. It was the same when I turned professional. I got to the top much faster than my contemporaries, even people like Simon Parke who was just as talented as I was.

Had I allowed myself to get things out of proportion? I thought back to the last long-term relationship I had had with a girlfriend. It had ended five years earlier when I was 22, long before my illness. There had been no one serious since then. Perhaps it was just that the right person hadn't come along, but then, perhaps I had been too focused on my squash career to notice if they had. When I got CFS I remember thinking that, as I didn't feel mentally fit, it might be better to steer clear of relationships for a while. I needed to concentrate on squash. At the time, that seemed a good decision for the sake of my career. Now I wasn't so sure. Perhaps it had not been a good decision from the perspective of being a fully rounded person.

It was good to think things through in this way, but in the end it was all speculation. There could be no definite conclusions, because there was no proof one way or another. Perhaps my illness had something to do with being driven to succeed; perhaps there was no connection at all. After all, lots of people are ambitious in their particular field yet don't become ill. Nevertheless, I felt this was interesting territory. It continued to occupy my mind for several months.

It was now approaching Christmas, and from then until February 1999 was a very hard time for me. I was trying to move forward, but constantly found my spirit being dragged down by the frustration of what had happened to me. Four years travelling all over the country and sometimes into Europe and America, seeing doctor after doctor, expert after expert, had yielded nothing at all. All this time I had been almost religious in my determination to do everything right in order to get well again. I had followed all the medical advice, taken all the right pills, eaten all the right foods, done the right amount of exercise and taken the prescribed amount of rest. None of it had worked. I was as badly off now as I had been at the start.

It seemed that CFS had won and there was nothing I could do about it. I had gone past the stage of feeling down and low. I now felt nothing at all. I had just become numb. There was no emotion left at all. It was a lonely and uncomfortable sensation. That was how I came to be out in the pubs in Nottingham city centre one night with friends. I had gone past caring, and decided to go out and enjoy myself. I must have had eight or nine pints of lager, a colossal amount for me. I had never been much of a drinker, although I had enjoyed winding down with friends and other players at the end of tournaments. After I became ill, I drank even less because chronic fatigue lowers your alcohol tolerance. The hangovers can last days or even weeks. I couldn't risk that kind of interruption while I was trying to get better, so I steered clear of drink. Now, it didn't seem to matter. My friends were surprised, of course – they were used to seeing me sipping fruit juices or making a couple of half-pints last the night. The vision of me knocking back pint after pint amused them at first. At last, Peter was letting his hair down. Whatever next! Behind the smiles, though, I think some of them were a little concerned and wondered what it meant. I didn't care at that point. I had given up hope. It was a big burden off my shoulders. As I drank, I felt elated.

After years of trying to be professional and highly disciplined, there was something strangely attractive about going to the opposite extreme and doing everything wrong. It was frustration, really. I had tried so many things and none of them had worked. I ended up going the other way and making myself worse. It was like throwing myself away. To most people a few drinks too many would be insignificant, but to me it was a major rebellion. I revelled in it. I could be silly and irresponsible like anybody else. It felt good. I wouldn't call it happiness, exactly, but it was the best I had felt for years. It didn't last long. I had another two nights on the town that week, but that was it. It wasn't really me; I knew that all along, but it did provide a brief escape from the frustration.

I didn't want to try any more treatments. In any case, there didn't seem to be much left to try except therapies that were on the very fringes. Cannabis was said to relieve symptoms for some people. Others had claimed benefits from royal jelly, extracts from the leaves of the ginkgo biloba trees or increasing the intake of trace elements like zinc or selenium. I glanced through them all, but they just confirmed my growing scepticism. I wasn't interested. I had had enough.

My experience with CFS had made me look at the body and medicine in a different light. It demonstrated that the medical world couldn't explain everything. It was baffled by CFS. So was I, but there was at least one thing I knew for certain; there was no one out there who was going to find the solution for me. Whatever the answer was, it was something I had to find out myself.

# 9

# WINNING THE WORLD CUP

Representing your country in a world cup is a big challenge at the best of times. When you haven't played a competitive match for two years, the task is even more daunting. It was a huge surprise and a great honour to be asked. I was desperate to play, but what if I let people down?

The England coach Dave Pearson told me not to worry. He had faith in my ability, even though I had been out of the game for so long. I told him I didn't know whether I would be able to play all the games required through the various rounds. He said it didn't matter. I could play as many or as few games as I wanted. He could not have been more supportive. I was moved that he was showing such confidence in me, but I was still uncertain about what to do. It's one thing to lose when you're playing purely for yourself; it's quite another to lose if it means letting down your team-mates and your country.

I sat back to consider what to do. It was hard to take it all in. The idea of being asked to play for England would have seemed unbelievable six months earlier, when I was feeling lost and bewildered with nowhere to turn. If someone had even suggested it as a possibility, I would have laughed at them. Yet now, fantastic though it seemed, it was really happening. It highlighted the incredible transformation I had gone through since that dark and depressing time, when I had been overcome by an overwhelming feeling of helplessness. That had been one of the worst periods of my life. My feelings were disorientating and made me behave in a way that was out of character. What did I think I was doing during those months? It just wasn't like me to give in to negative thoughts. I had always been a fighter; it was one of the main ways I defined myself. That sudden descent into despair wasn't me at all. It wasn't part of my make-up to crumble.

What was it all about? I had no idea at the time. I'm still not sure, but perhaps it was all part of the healing process. Maybe I had to hit rock bottom before I could start building myself up again. The first big hurdle was coming to terms with the fact that I would probably never know for certain what was wrong with me. After years of soul-searching and listening to countless experts, I was no closer to finding an answer. That was depressing in itself. It's traumatic enough to suffer from a debilitating illness that plays havoc with your life and destroys your career, but the fact that no one can explain it makes it even more difficult to bear.

Despite the lack of medical knowledge and proper research, I had pressed on for four years hoping against hope that somehow I would find an explanation for what was going on in my body. Then, at some point during those months of despair, I'm not sure exactly when, I think I finally came to terms with the fact that I would never find such an explanation. At least, not in the near future; certainly not in time for it to have any positive effect on my career.

In a strange way, it was a relief to admit that I wasn't going to find the answers I had been seeking. It took away the pressure of constantly agonising over what I should try next. Life became more simple. There was no need to do anything, no need to try anything. Nothing worked. Medical science was beaten and so, therefore, was I. It's not as if I didn't have my own ideas. You can't spend five years fighting something without forming a theory about what you're up against. I believed that no one could explain CFS because of the dual nature of the illness. It's caused by a combination of both physical and psychological factors. To treat it, you have to look at the whole person and their lifestyle. That's why the medical world hadn't even come close to finding a cure. There is no single drug that will make both the body and the mind feel better. You have to take a broader approach.

I didn't know why I got CFS, but from a physical point of view I was sure it had a lot to do with the bout of glandular fever. That part, at least, was textbook stuff. Glandular fever is caused by the Epstein-Barr virus, something that is found in many CFS sufferers. In some way, I felt this had weakened my immune system which left me prone to more viral infections. Of course, it may have been the other way round. There might have always been a problem with my immune system, which would explain why I got glandular fever in the first place, why I suffered repeatedly from tonsillitis as a child and then endured endless colds and bouts of flu as an adult. People who think CFS is all in the mind should take these things into account. I have no doubt that CFS has a physical cause.

On the other hand, I also believe that psychological factors can play a significant part. Not all glandular fever sufferers go on to develop CFS. There must have been something else, something to do with me as an individual. I came to suspect that the mental strength on which I prided myself may have played a large part in my downfall. I was so driven that even when I was recovering from glandular fever I was determined to carry on training and working when perhaps I should have stopped. This continued over the following years, right up to the final of the British Open.

I had the mental strength to push on no matter how tired I felt. I was able to drag myself on to the squash court to practise and go through rigorous training schedules, even though I felt mentally and physically exhausted. I was able to psych myself up to travel thousands of miles to tournaments and battle through to the finals even though my body was crying out for rest. It was something I felt I had to do to achieve my goal. In the end, however, perhaps it had been counter-productive. My strength became my weakness, and eventually my body could take no more. Perhaps it had some inbuilt safety mechanism that shut itself down and refused to let me continue. At least, that's what I thought had happened. I realised that lots of people push themselves hard and they don't get CFS. No one was more driven than Jonah Barrington. He had enormous willpower and determination. He too forced himself on when his body was screaming for rest, but he didn't develop CFS. On the other hand, he had never had anything like glandular fever. It seemed reasonable to conclude that the glandular fever had weakened me in some way; perhaps it weakens lots of people, but they don't notice it because they don't drive themselves like I had. I might not have noticed it if I hadn't pushed myself as hard as I did.

The explanation had a certain neatness, and at least took into account both the physical and psychological nature of the illness. I didn't regard it as conclusive, however. I had no proof and it was just a theory with little scientific research to back it up; just my own experiences. I knew it was entirely possible that I was wrong and the real cause was something yet to be discovered. On the other hand, my explanation made as much sense as any other I had come across.

As you might imagine, I agonised over these points for hours on end without ever getting anywhere. During those months of despair I had very little else to do. Every day I looked back over what had happened to me, asking myself how I might have done things differently. Part of me berated myself for not having rested when I was feeling ill. How could I have been so shortsighted? But then I would ask myself what I was supposed to have done, given the lack of knowledge about my condition. If it had been something definite like hepatitis, I would have had no trouble allowing myself time to recover. I would have been much more relaxed because I wouldn't have been wondering whether I should be playing instead of resting. I would have gone on holiday for six months and forgotten about squash.

As it was, I had done all I could in the circumstances. I had been to see numerous doctors who all did blood tests and a hundred and one other things, and told me there was nothing wrong with me. In those circumstances, what are you supposed to do except try to pull yourself together and get on with things? I wasn't stupid. If some doctor could have done a test and told me I had such-and-such an illness which required me to do this, this and this in order to get well then I would have followed that advice to the letter. Unfortunately, no one was giving me any such advice. No one could, because no one knew what to do.

Even when my CFS was diagnosed two years after I first became ill, there were still conflicting opinions as to how to deal with it. Most doctors advocated rest, but others disagreed, putting doubts into my mind. As I lay at home trying to take things easy, there was always part of me thinking that perhaps I should try to brush aside my problems and get back to work. That, together with my anxiety about my career and the fact that I was losing so much ground, meant that I never really rested properly. My body may have been taking it easy but my mind was still working overtime. It was worrying about how much I was missing out on and whether I would ever be able to get back to where I was before. Apart from my career, I was anxious about my health and whether I could ever look forward to a time when I would stop feeling exhausted. It meant I was probably going through as much if not more nervous energy than I had been before I became ill. There could be no real rest under those circumstances. That's why the months doing nothing didn't make me feel any better.

With something so uncertain as CFS, you find yourself going round in circles without ever being able to reach a definite conclusion that you can accept and which provides any real help. You can only analyse for so long before you have to accept that you aren't getting anywhere and it's time to let it pass. This isn't a conclusion you come to easily or quickly, but eventually it's forced upon you because there is nowhere else to go. By about March 1999, I had reached that point. I had tried all the supposed cures and examined all the latest theories and was no better off. Now I was ready to stop all the agonising. I was finally coming to terms with my situation. I stopped trying to rationalise it and started to accept it. In a strange way, it was a great release. I think I felt better just for that.

I then decided to get away from it all and took three holidays one after another. I went to Marbella with a girlfriend, and then visited my parents on their boat. I remember talking to my dad and telling him that I wasn't sure if I could play anymore. I said I was tired of trying and the effort was getting too much. I think he felt that I ought to stop playing, but he didn't really want to say it. He was trying to find the words to hint that maybe the time had come to move on and do something new. I knew he would support me whatever I did and I continued wondering what to do for the best.

I was still wondering when I went on yet another holiday to Portugal with Simon Parke and his girlfriend. I had a great time and felt more relaxed than I had for a long time. Then one evening when I was speaking to Simon I surprised myself by suddenly blurting out that I didn't think I would ever play again. I didn't see any way back – I might as well accept it and get on with the rest of my life. This was a huge leap for me. I had expressed doubts to my dad a few weeks earlier, but was trying to tell myself that I would be back playing before long. At the time I had believed that, but now I felt as if it was all just a pipedream.

In some ways, the whole experience of my illness seemed like a dream. There were times when I almost believed it hadn't really happened to me at all. I half expected to wake up and find out that none of it was true. It's hard to come to terms with something when part of you is thinking: 'Is this really happening to me?' But it was happening, all right. Unfortunately, there was no waking up to come; no happy conclusion when I realised it had all been only a nightmare. I had done all I could and it was time to be philosophical about things. I had to accept reality. Simon seemed surprised, but he didn't try to dissuade me. He knew how much it meant to me to start playing again, and he realised I wouldn't say such things if I didn't mean them. He just said that if I was feeling like that then it was probably the best thing to do.

We didn't talk about it any more after that, but I felt better for just acknowledging what seemed to be the inevitable. By finally allowing myself to say 'That's it. I'm going to stop,' I took an enormous amount of pressure off myself. It was similar to the relief I had felt when I gave up trying to find an explanation for my condition. Now I had reached a stage where I accepted there was no more I could do about any of it except put it all behind me and get on with something new. In many ways, it was an exciting prospect. It was certainly a release, a letting go. There was no need to worry any more. I felt better for having such a burden removed from my shoulders. I lay back to enjoy the sunshine and the rest of the holiday. It felt good. I was more at peace than I had been for years.

I came back from those holidays feeling much better mentally. I was no longer worrying myself over things I couldn't control, and had come to terms with the fact that my career was as good as over. The only question was what to do next. Although I now felt much more relaxed about things and therefore much better generally, I still felt physically weak and couldn't concentrate well for long periods without getting tired. The symptoms of CFS were still there. Nevertheless, I felt confident enough to start thinking again about treatments that might help me now that I had found a new sense of peace.

About a year earlier, I had read a CFS newsletter discussing the benefits of Phenelzine, the drug I had tried that caused so many unpleasant side effects. A doctor was quoted as saying he had achieved a lot of success by prescribing small doses to some of his patients. The dosage he mentioned was much lower than the amount I had taken. This seemed interesting, if not convincing, and I wondered about whether I ought to try it. Perhaps it was time to give the medical world another chance. I was planning to visit my sister in London at the time, and it turned out that she lived close to the hospital where this doctor worked. I called in to see him and told him the whole story of what had happened. I described the adverse effects that Phenelzine had caused before. He advised me to try again, but with only a quarter of the dose I had been taking before. I agreed, although I wasn't expecting anything dramatic to happen.

To my surprise, however, I did start to feel better physically. It wasn't a dramatic improvement by any means, but it was a step in the right direction. The fact that there was an improvement at all was enough to raise my spirits a bit, and that in turn made me feel even stronger. I felt I was getting a virtuous circle going, with the mental and the physical drawing impetus from each other.

During the next few weeks, my health improved faster than at any other period since I had first become ill. It was all very encouraging, but I had been through too much and had had too many disappointments to get over-excited. I continued resting and taking the tablets, and kept making progress. Unlike before, with the higher dosage, there weren't any side effects. Soon, I felt strong enough to do a bit more exercise and started to go back on court. It wasn't with a view to resurrecting my career; I just wanted to enjoy having a knock around and start to get fit again, in the way that anyone might want to do. This was probably significant because it was the first time since I had become ill that I had started playing without hoping that I would soon be able to get back to normal. I no longer had any expectation of ever playing again professionally. It meant I didn't feel any pressure to perform. I felt very relaxed, and was simply enjoying the fact that I didn't feel exhausted every time I went on court for a gentle knock around.

It was quite a revelation, really. I had forgotten how much I actually enjoyed playing squash. Once you become a professional, it ceases to be something you do simply for fun. You enjoy it, of course, but it's your work and for much of the time that's how it feels. You don't think about it as being your hobby and a leisure activity. I was starting to think of it like that again, however, and it felt good. Several weeks passed with me gradually doing more and more on court without feeling any ill effects. I trained a bit harder and started growing in confidence. I was beginning to feel good. After all those years of struggling, it was exhilarating to play and exercise and to come off court feeling fine and looking forward to the next session.

After a while, I felt so positive that I arranged a game against Simon Parke, just for fun. That soon put me in my place. He blasted me off court without even trying. I didn't care, though. The thrashing did nothing to dent my growing confidence, because I still felt fine. I was obviously yards off the pace of the game, and I had nothing like the necessary fitness to compete against him, but it didn't matter. I had played a full game and come through it unscathed. I stepped up my training without any ill effects. I continued playing Simon and continued to get thrashed, but at least the margin was narrowing a little.

Soon, I began to wonder if making another comeback might be a possibility after all. I thought it was unlikely, but saw no harm in continuing to build up my fitness. My thinking was now very different from the way it had been in the past; I had no illusions and no great expectations, and I think that probably helped me. I was more stoical about everything. I realised the odds were against me and that was fine. If this turned out to be just another false dawn I would be able to cope with it. I was still taking the Phenelzine, which was proving very effective as an energiser, but I realised that my state of mind was equally, if not more, important to my wellbeing. Although I was feeling better, it was almost certain that the CFS was still in my system. There had been no big breakthrough and no sudden cure to suggest otherwise.

The issue at that stage, therefore, was not how to get rid of the CFS but how well I could control it. I was sure that coming to terms with the likelihood of not playing again had taken a lot of pressure off me and was probably the first step towards feeling better. I didn't want to fall into the trap of putting that pressure back on to myself by hoping too much that I might make a comeback now. In all honesty, I think I had reached a stage where it genuinely didn't matter too much. I pressed on at a steady pace. My strength was growing by the day, but I wasn't going to make any assumptions. If I could get back to playing again that would be fine. If I couldn't, then I could cope with it. I would be no worse off than I was before.

Everything continued to go well for me right into June. I was training harder, practising more and there were no signs of any ill effects. I felt strong enough to train again with the England squad. Again, it was nothing too serious. I was taking one step at a time and seeing how I felt after each one. It was going well. The other players could beat me fairly easily but the thrashings weren't quite as convincing as that first game against Simon a few months earlier. After a few weeks, they were still beating me but the thrashings had stopped. I was getting closer every day and instead of feeling weakened, I could sense myself getting stronger. Soon I was able to give the others a decent game and make them work a bit. Before much longer, I was taking games off them and starting to compete on level terms.

It was great to be back playing again and using the competitive side of my nature. It did a great deal for my self-esteem. When I became ill and unable to play any more, it was almost like being thrown out of work. Now I felt good because I was able to do my job again and my confidence grew. I was amazed and delighted that I was able to return to such a good standard in such a short space of time. I think it helped that I had never let myself go throughout my illness, no matter how badly I felt. I never put on any weight and apart from the times when I was particularly ill and weak, I had always tried to do a little exercise. Often this had been going on court by myself and knocking the ball about. It was honing technique rather than trying to play or do any physical training. This turned out to be a great advantage because when I did start playing again, my skill level hadn't dropped all that far and it wasn't that hard to get it back. I think I was also helped by the fact that I had played since I was about six or seven. Skills learnt in childhood stay with you for a long time; probably much longer than anything learnt as an adult.

Physical strength was another matter. I was still a long way off my peak fitness and knew it would take several months, if not a year, to get back to where I had once been. Nevertheless, I had come a long way in only a few months. It was exhilarating to feel myself getting stronger every day, but I wasn't going to let myself get carried away. It was one thing to train with the top players and do reasonably well against them; it was another matter entirely to play competitively in serious matches. Nevertheless, I was doing well enough to start thinking that maybe I could make another return and see how I got on. I had made tremendous progress without really trying. If I could continue to get stronger and work on my style of play so that it was less physically demanding, then maybe it wasn't out of the question.

I knew I would have to move cautiously. The last thing I wanted was a relapse. Just the thought of falling ill stopped me in my tracks and made me think. Did I really want to risk another breakdown? And what if I couldn't do it anyway? How did I know the other England players weren't just going easy on me? After all, how would I react if I were playing a guy who'd been ill for four years? I would hardly want to humiliate him. I would give him an easy time. Maybe that's what they were doing with me. Perhaps my sudden return to form wasn't as real as I had imagined.

These and several other doubts fluttered around my mind, and there was still a part of me that thought a comeback was a bad idea. Then came that call from Dave Pearson. He phoned me up out of the blue and said: 'Would you be prepared to play for England in the World Cup if you were selected?' I was totally taken aback, but said that of course I would, if I felt I could do all right. Every player wants to represent his country. I told him of my doubts. I wasn't sure if it was right for me to go back into the game, or if I was still good enough and, more importantly, strong enough to compete at the top level. Dave told me he was sure that I could. He seemed very positive and enthusiastic about the idea, which gave me a lot of confidence. If someone shows faith in you to the point where they're prepared to throw you in at the deep end in an international match, it's bound to give you a boost.

The offer set my mind racing. Could I really come back and do it again? Why not? I had done it two years earlier, but my health let me down that time. I felt better now, but who was to say I wouldn't break down again? And what if I couldn't carry on playing and let the team down? Dave told me not to worry. He said I didn't have to play every match. If I wanted, I could just play the quarter-finals or perhaps the semis. I could do as much or as little as I wanted. It was a fantastic gesture of support on his part and I really appreciated it. The offer suited me more than it did the team, really. I didn't want to mislead anyone. I said I probably wouldn't be able to play three games on the trot. I might only be able to play one and then have to miss the rest of the tournament. He said: 'That's fine. Anything as long as it gets you playing again.'

Well, offers that generous don't come along every day. It was hard to say no. Dave's support was very welcome, but it was not without some risk on his part. English squash benefits from lottery support, but it has to be earned by success on the court. To qualify for the full amount, the England camp has to get so many players in the top ten, so many in the top twenty and so on. It has to show significant development of young players and a growing support for the game at grass roots level. It's a major undertaking, and there's a great deal of money to be lost if they get things wrong. Dave and the rest of the England set-up were looking for players who could get into the world top ten and help fulfil the lottery requirements. They obviously thought I had the potential to do that for them because I had a proven track record. I had been there before, all the way up to number two. The only thing that had stopped me was my health and if that was showing signs of improving, they wanted to encourage me because they thought I could do well. That would be good not only for me, but also for the finances of the game. However, if I were to fail it could jeopardise the amount of money they would get from the lottery commission. They were perhaps encouraged to look at me because although England had top players like Simon Parke, Paul Johnson and Chris Walker, there weren't many good younger players coming through.

Apart from wanting to compete for my own sake, I wanted to play as a way of repaying the support shown me by the England set-up since my failed comeback attempt two years earlier. I had also received some money from the lottery fund, which had helped me to keep going when the insurance money stopped. That money had obviously been paid in the hope that I would one day return and put something back into the game. Helping England to win the World Cup would go some way towards doing that. I was torn between wanting to help the team and being worried about letting them down.

I decided to go for it. If they had faith in me then the least I could do was have faith in myself. I started to train harder over the summer and made good progress. I still wasn't anywhere near my peak when the tournament began in August, but I had done as much as I could. I consoled myself with the knowledge that I didn't have to play every game and could pull out at any time. I came into the tournament at the semi-final stage. Although I felt a little nervous, it was good to be back on court in full competitive games again. I need not have worried. I was a bit rusty at first, but I won all my three matches. Two of them were against top ranking players.

David Evans of Wales had emerged at the top level after I had stopped playing. He was ranked in the top twenty when we finally met. It was a great test for me; he was a very good player, as his high ranking suggested. I felt relaxed once the game got started. In a way, the pressure was on him because I had been out for so long. Also, I probably had the advantage of being fresher and keener. People who've been playing day in and day out on the circuit can get a bit stale and lose some of their edge. For me, it was like playing my first professional match again and that was very powerful. I won relatively easily. It was a great feeling to know that I could still perform at that level.

The next day I came up against an old adversary, Rodney Eyles. He was still ranked in the world top twenty and had been world champion only two years before. It was my third game in three days, but I still felt reasonably strong. The score was 1–1 with Australia, so I was playing the deciding game, which put more pressure on me. I enjoyed every minute of it and won 3–0.

It was fantastic to be back and able to compete against such strong opposition. Just to have put up a good performance would have been a great boost for me, but to win all three matches was almost too good to be true. I felt a bit tired after the three games in three days so they decided against risking me in the final. I was fine with that. I was delighted just to be there. In any case, the team were more than able to cope without me. England beat Scotland in the final and it was great to be there to cheer them on, even more so as I had been a part of the victory. Perhaps I could find a way back after all.

# 10.
## THE BIGGER PICTURE

The World Cup victory was a terrific boost and set my mind racing. It was no longer a case of could I make a comeback, but when and how. I had been through too much to get carried away, however. I was sure the CFS was still lurking in my system ready to strike me down at any time. My only chance was to work out a way of managing it. If I was going to return to the circuit I would have to do it properly, taking my illness into account. The last thing I wanted was another abortive comeback attempt. I was confident, however, that things would be different this time. I was older, wiser and much stronger, both physically and mentally.

There were still a lot of potential pitfalls along the way, but I felt I had learnt how to deal with them. I knew that I would have to take a long-term view and build up gradually, even if that were to prove frustrating at times. It would pay dividends in the long run by making my return more sustainable. I had already paved the way by building up my fitness over a five-month period – much longer than for my first comeback attempt two years earlier – and I felt all the stronger for it.

There was, of course, a lot more to it than making sure I didn't overtrain or rush into tournaments too soon. My attitude would have to change. I wanted to be more relaxed and not allow everything to matter too much to me. As I had discovered, and Dr Budgett had pointed out, it wasn't just the physical exertion that caused problems, although they were real enough. The stress and pressure of competing in the big tournaments could be just as draining. I knew I would be just as competitive as ever. There would be no point in playing otherwise, but I could help myself by limiting the number of events I entered until I felt stronger. It was also vital to make sure I got plenty of rest, even if it meant missing training sessions. It would be better to go into tournaments lacking a little fitness than to be overtrained and exhausted. At the first sign of trouble, I would rest and wait until I felt better before trying anything again.

By changing the way I played, I felt, I could help myself a lot. Before I became ill, my game had been very physical. That approach was unlikely to suit me now. After all I had been through I didn't want to be playing long, hard matches if I could help it. I wanted to improve tactically and be able to play winning shots earlier in the rally. If you can play the better quality squash, then you can get your opponent on the run and make him do all the hard work. It means that even if he's fitter than you are he's likely to tire first, because he's using up more energy. All the skills work I had done when I was ill had helped me a little with this. My touch was probably better than ever. I had also had a lot of time to think about the game and watch other players in action. I was probably more tactically aware than I had ever been. However, I was well aware that while my plans might be all very well in theory, it would be quite another matter to put them into practice. There was only one way to find out. I had to get back out there on the circuit and get on with it.

The bad news was that I would have to do it the hard way. I was no longer Peter Marshall the world number two and heir apparent to Jansher Khan. I was now outside the world rankings and so had no automatic right to compete in the top tournaments. I would have to take my chances with all the young hopefuls and earn my place in the qualifying rounds. This made things a lot more difficult. I was now confident that I could beat anyone in a one-off game. The question was whether I was strong enough to keep going over a whole tournament. That had been my problem before. Having to play two or three qualifying matches added to the burden, and gave the top seeds I would eventually have to face yet another advantage over me.

I decided to play only in world ranking tournaments at first so I could start moving up the ladder as quickly as possible. If I did well it might only take five or six tournaments to get back into the top 24, and then I wouldn't have to qualify any more. I was determined to assess how I felt after each tournament and not play again until I was sure that I had fully recovered, even if it meant sitting out some of the main events of the year. It was important for me to retain control and not start feeling driven again. That approach could only lead to more problems. I was 28 at the time, and if I was careful I could reasonably expect to get another four years out of the game. The only way to do this was to look at the bigger picture and sacrifice short-term expediency for long-term benefit.

The World Open in Egypt was the first big tournament coming up that I could enter. I got through the first qualifying round, but injured my back in the second match and had to withdraw. The irony wasn't lost on me. After four years fighting CFS, I was finally starting to see some light at the end of the tunnel only to have it snuffed out by a mundane injury. It wasn't surprising really, considering that I hadn't played for a long time or done much training. My muscles and ligaments weren't used to being pushed and would take time to regain their strength and suppleness. I was out for two weeks.

There was nothing I could do but make the most of my unexpected rest period. When Martin Heath got knocked out of the tournament, he suggested catching a bus to the shores of the Red Sea to spend a few days snorkelling. It seemed a great idea and I agreed straight away. When we got to the coast, I changed $300 into Egyptian currency and put it into my rucksack. Martin watched me and then started laughing. He asked why I hadn't folded the money up and put it away carefully in a wallet as anyone else would. Apparently, my mind was on something else and I had just crumpled up the notes and stuffed them in the bag along with my passport. I didn't really have an answer. He gave me one of his quizzical looks, as if marvelling at my lack of basic life skills. I thought no more about it and set off walking to the beach.

After a few minutes, I realised that Martin was still chuckling away to himself behind me. I turned round to see him holding a fistful of Egyptian notes. They had fallen out of my bag because the zip was broken. I hadn't realised. Martin had been picking them up one by one as they fell out, trying not to laugh so he could see how far I would get before I caught on. He told me my CFS might be better, but I was as absent-minded as ever! 'Why do you have such a total disregard for things other people would consider important, like money?' he asked. 'Or is it that maybe you just have too much?' I assured him that, after four years out of the game, that was most certainly not the case. He just kept shaking his head, asking himself how I ever managed to get from one place to another.

I managed to hold on to my money for the rest of the trip, and we had a very relaxing time, snorkelling and sunbathing. Fortunately, my back injury recovered just in time for me to enter the Detroit Open. It was nothing like as grand as the World Open, but it was a starting point. There were some advantages to beginning with a smaller event: it was largely ignored by the world's top ten players so it would provide a relatively gentle return to the circuit. It would also give me the chance to earn some desperately needed world ranking points.

Having said that, however, it wasn't going to be easy. Most of the players ranked between ten and thirty in the world were taking part. They would all be keen to break into the top ten and would be giving it everything they'd got. I also had to be careful not to get too far ahead of myself. Before I started worrying about how to beat the high-ranking players, I first had to qualify. That would take three matches before I even got into the tournament proper. Nothing could be taken for granted.

I flew out to Detroit and although on one level I was very confident, there was a part of me that was very nervous. I had doubts and was questioning myself all the time. When it comes to the crunch, no one is 100 per cent confident of their ability. I certainly wasn't. I took comfort from my performances in the World Cup, but I knew that playing well over a full tournament was another matter. I still wondered what level I was really at and whether I could get back a truly high standard; just as important, could I maintain that standard match after match? I drew on all my experience from my earlier playing days to give me the confidence I needed. This was only partly successful, however, because my achievements before my illness couldn't tell me much about how I would perform now.

In the qualifying rounds, I came up against the very talented young Australian player, Anthony Ricketts. I hadn't met him before and so neither of us really knew what to expect. I don't know how he felt, but I was very nervous. I tried to concentrate on using my new economical game plan and make my opponent do most of the work, but I wasn't all that successful. As soon as the game got under way, I found I had little time to think and did what all players do when the pressure is really on; I reverted to type and started playing by instinct. This meant the hard, fast pace game that I had used successfully in the early part of my career. The problem was that I no longer had the strength and fitness to employ it quite so successfully.

It turned out to be a very long and tough game. I wasn't match sharp and I didn't play very well. I found myself just grinding it out. Although I eventually won 3–2, I wasn't happy with the way I had played. There wasn't much quality in my game and I had to rely too much on adrenaline and determination. It was a relief to get through it but I came off court wondering how I would react physically after such a draining game. It was the last thing I needed. I didn't feel too tired as I rested that evening, but I remember thinking that I probably wouldn't progress much further after such a tough start. I was pleased to have won but I knew I wouldn't be happy if that was going to be my level for the future. I wondered if I had more to give and drifted off to sleep not sure of the answer.

Thankfully, the next qualifying game was a lot easier and I won 3–0. After that, I seemed to get better and better. I made it through to the main draw and came up against Paul Price in the first round. He was ranked number 12 in the world and went on to get into the top ten. Within a year, he was to reach the final of the game's most prestigious tournament, the British Open. I beat him 3–0 and could sense the improvement in the way I was playing. I had a tough match against Lee Beachill the following day, including two physically draining games which both went to 17–15 scores. I always felt on top, however, and came through 3–1. Graham Ryding withdrew injured in the semi-final when I was 2–0 up so I was through to the final. That brought me up against another very talented top 20 player, David Palmer. Again, I won 3–0 and felt comfortable all the way.

I had got my first tournament win for five years. It was a relief. I had done much better than I had expected after that tough opening game against Anthony Ricketts. As I looked back at the tournament, I felt that game was probably something of a turning point for me. It was very close and if I had lost it would have knocked my confidence. As it was, I only just scraped through but that was enough. It got me started and as the tournament went on I started to move a lot better and was able to hit the ball more cleanly. You can only really make these improvements when you're out there competing against the top players. No amount of training can compensate for lack of match practice. I felt I had probably responded better than I could have expected. I was also very encouraged by the fact that I had played six matches in six days and come through it unscathed.

The ability to compete day after day would be vital if I was going to have a realistic chance of getting back to the top.

It was fantastic to win, but it was also a great feeling just to be there and savour the atmosphere of the squash circuit again. It was strange at first. I would be warming up for a game and odd memories would come back to me of former matches and their triumphs and failures. I kept meeting people I had known before which was really good, but probably the most startling thing for me was the number of people I didn't know. The whole circuit seemed to have changed in the four years I had been out. There were a lot of young players about and I felt a bit of a senior citizen among them.

Lee Beachill was only a junior when I stopped playing, and now he was an established pro. It was the same with most of the other players there and it made for an interesting contrast. I didn't know what to expect from them and I suppose they didn't know what to expect from me. They had probably heard about me and may have seen me play, but had never played me themselves. They couldn't be sure how I would perform. I might go on court feeling tired and suffering the effects of my long lay-off, or they might meet me on the day when everything clicked and came right for me. I was an unknown quantity and I think that made it hard for my opponents.

The uncertainty added to the excitement I felt to be back playing. It was like when I was a youngster starting out for the first time. Everything was new and different. Most players quickly get used to the daily grind and want to get away from it as soon as they come off court, but I wanted to savour every moment of the tournament. When I finished playing, I stayed on to watch the other matches just as I had when I started on the circuit. When you're a newcomer, you want to sample everything. I knew that feeling would wear off after I had played a few more tournaments, but it's good while it lasts. That extra freshness you feel can take you a long way. You see a lot of youngsters who do well for a while because they're enjoying themselves so much, yet fade a little later on when the excitement wanes and they find it harder to motivate themselves.

Being back on the circuit meant a return to travelling and living out of a suitcase but I didn't mind that. After so long cooped up at home, it was good to get away and travel. I appreciated it much more this time because

I was older. I stayed with a family in Detroit rather than put up with the blandness of the hotel. It was much better, because they took the time to show me around and I was keen to see the sights and enjoy the overall experience.

I knew I couldn't be sure how the tournament had affected me until several days after it had ended. I felt great immediately after the final but, of course, at that time I was pumped up on excitement and adrenaline which would mask any tiredness I might feel. I was okay for a while, but a few days afterwards I started to feel more and more drained. It was nothing dramatic, but I wanted to monitor the situation very carefully. I could tell the difference between ordinary tiredness linked to a lot of hard work and the tiredness associated with my illness. With the onset of CFS I would feel as though I was getting flu and I would want to sleep all the time; ten hours at night and then two or three hours in the day. I might have a sore throat and my glands might swell a bit. I would often feel down mentally as well. Ordinary tiredness from matchplay was much more specific; just heavy muscles which had been put through their paces. The recovery rate was very quick; little more than a day or two.

A few more days passed and I still wasn't 100 per cent right. It didn't really feel as though CFS was returning, and the fatigue was perhaps no more than the reaction you might expect, having played a tournament when you've been out of the game so long. I couldn't be sure and had to decide what to do next. I was due to play another medium-sized tournament in Chicago the following week. I felt I would probably be all right but after thinking about it carefully, I decided to withdraw. I wasn't particularly worried, but thought it wise to err on the side of caution. I was determined to avoid the mistakes I had made before by doing too much too soon. I didn't want to submit myself to the rigours of a tournament unless I felt fully fit. If I started the first match feeling tired, I might deteriorate rapidly the more games I played. I wanted to avoid any cumulative descent into CFS again.

It was disappointing in a way to pull out when I had got some momentum going, but I knew I had to be tough with myself and stick to my strategy of a careful return. Instead of going to Chicago, I went to Boston to stay with an old friend from Millfield called Angus Kirkland, now a professional squash coach. I had a good time relaxing with him and his family. I did nothing for ten days except rest. There was no training, no playing and I tried to think about the game as little as possible. It was a big departure from my previous approach, when I tried to make a comeback two years earlier. Then I would almost certainly have played Chicago and may have done myself more harm than good.

Now I was more experienced. I could recognise the early symptoms of CFS and I didn't want to take any chances. There was a balance to be struck, of course. Too much resting can knock your fitness but, again, I had learnt from experience that I could get that back quite quickly. I returned home to Nottingham and continued to take it easy, although I started going back on court for a few sessions. I felt fine. Whether that was because of the rest I had taken or whether I would have been all right anyway I can't say, but I was pleased that I had stuck to my strategy of a gradual return.

The question was what to do next. I needed more tournaments but it was hard to get into them. Before going to Detroit, I had looked at the possibility of playing the Pakistan Open. I had no chance. There were 24 automatic places for the top players and another eight places available to qualifiers. The problem was that only 32 players were eligible to compete in the qualifying rounds. It meant you had to be in the top 50 just to be able to enter. The win in Detroit had rocketed me from nowhere to 109 in the world. That was a great leap, but I was still a long way off. Fortunately for me, somebody pulled out of the qualifying rounds, leaving a spare space. I was invited to enter. It was a great opportunity to get more tournament practice and earn some ranking points.

The Pakistan Open was an unusual tournament in some ways. Pakistan is one of the strongest squash nations in the world, both in terms of the quality of its players and the amount of support the game receives. Despite this, the country's major tournament is not one of the game's top events. This is partly because the prize money isn't that high, but it's also to do with the fact that Karachi is such a long trek. Many of the top players don't compete because they don't like the idea of the journey nor the hot, humid conditions when they get there. Those things didn't bother me at all. I was just grateful to be able to take part in the tournament. The fact that most of the world's top ten would be absent increased my chances of doing well and moving up the rankings. Having said that, I knew the overall standard would be higher than in Detroit.

Up to that point, the Pakistan Open was unique in its list of champions. In its 15-year history, only one surname had ever appeared on the winner's trophy: that of Khan. First it was Jahingir Khan, then Jansher and finally the latest in the dynasty, Amjad. They were all spurred on to victory by the loud and passionate home support. Foreign challengers had come and gone but no one had ever got a look-in.

If anything was going to prove to myself and others that I was really back in business, it was success in the sweltering heat of Karachi. I needed to be in good condition to do it but I was also determined not to fall into the trap of trying too hard. My health was more important to me than anything, so I continued to get plenty of rest as the tournament approached. I just played practice games and didn't worry too much about fitness training. I would save the big effort for the tournament.

One of the first people I bumped into when I got there was none other than Jahingir Khan. It was fantastic to see him again after all those years. We chatted for a while and he was very supportive. He thought it was unfair that I had to qualify for tournaments after losing my world ranking. He'd had a long period out of the game with a back injury at the end of his career, and when he wanted to come back he was in the same position as me and had to qualify. He was nearly 30 at the time and realised it could take him a year to get back to the top. By then, his powers might be starting to fade and he would start going down again. He didn't want to go through all that so he stopped playing. That was a big loss to the game.

Jahingir thought the rules ought to be changed to make it easier for top players to return after a long-term injury. In tennis, players are given a provisional ranking when they come back so they can start again where they left off. It only lasts a few months and it's up to them to justify it, but at least it gives them a chance. We talked over old times a little and the conversation soon got round to the standard of the modern players. Jahingir didn't think the standard was as high as when he was playing. I don't think it's a point he wanted to make too often in public; he feared it might sound like sour grapes, seeing as he had retired. He was able to say it to me, however, because I had been around when he was playing.

I agreed with him about the decline in standard at the very highest level. The top five at that time couldn't compare with the top five in the latter stages of Jahingir's career. However, I think it would be unfair to criticise the top players at the time for falling short of Jahingir's standards. He was playing during an exceptional period. He and Jansher were the two greatest players of all time. Closely following them were Rod Martin, Chris Dittmar and Chris Robertson. They would all have been undisputed number ones at most other periods of the game. Together, they were probably the best top five there has ever been. It wasn't only the modern players who would be second best to them; the top five from any era would be found wanting.

Ironically, while those players at the very top might not have been as formidable as the earlier stars, the overall standard of the game was much higher. For example, my first game at the Detroit Open was against the young Australian Anthony Ricketts. He was outside the top 50 at the time, yet he was an excellent player. There were no players of his standard that low down the rankings when I started out. It means that these days there are no easy games any more.

As I considered the improvement in overall standard, I realised that even qualifying for a tournament like the Pakistan Open could be difficult. Fortunately, I managed to get through and came up against Omar Elborolossy in the first round proper. I won 3–0. That sounds comfortable, but it was a tough game and I came close to losing it because I still lacked some strength. But somehow it kick-started me into action, and I had two 3–0 wins, more comfortable than the first, against another Egyptian, Amr Shabana, and then the Australian John Williams. I came up against Thierry Lincou from France in the semi-final. I was starting to feel tired at this point, not because of CFS but because I had played five matches in quick succession and wasn't used to it yet. It turned out to be the toughest game of the tournament, but I came through it 3–1.

I could hardly believe it. I was in the final. It was a fantastic feeling because it brought back so many memories for me. I had been to Pakistan a lot before I became ill, and always enjoyed playing there. It held so much history for me; I'd had many battles with Jansher, including that epic 3–2 battle in the 1994 final when I played some of the best squash of my life. Looking back on matches like that gave me inspiration. I automatically started to replay them in my mind. I couldn't believe I had the chance to play there in yet another final.

To add even more spice to the occasion, my opponent in the final was the title-holder, Amjad Khan, Jansher's nephew. The atmosphere on the day was fantastic. The crowd were very loud and boisterous. Everyone was cheering for Amjad, obviously, but I didn't mind that. My only concern was that so far it had been another tough tournament for me, and I wondered if I would have enough energy to perform well on the big occasion. I was hoping I wouldn't tire too quickly but was looking forward to it. It was wonderful just to be there. It was a huge event, as it always is in Pakistan. The final was being shown live on television.

The first thing I saw when I arrived at the court was Jansher's coach sitting in the same familiar corner he had occupied back in 1994. That certainly brought the memories flooding back. Everything seemed just the way it had been five years earlier. The only difference was that I was playing Amjad and not Jansher. No disrespect to Amjad, but he was a less daunting prospect. Even so, he turned out to be a tough opponent and took the first game quite easily. Thankfully, I was able to come back and take the match 3–1. It made quite a pleasant change to turn the tables on a member of the Khan family for once. It was a fantastic moment. I could hardly believe it; my second title in only my second tournament.

The Pakistani crowd were very supportive. They were obviously disappointed to see their local hero beaten, but were generous in their applause. I flew home with that applause still ringing in my ears. It had been a fantastic couple of months for me. I had won my first two tournaments. Most of my opponents had been seasoned professionals in the world top 20. It was very reassuring and proved I could still play at a very high level and sustain it over a whole tournament. I felt tired coming back from Pakistan, but not as bad as I had after Detroit, so I took comfort from that.

There was more confirmation of my progress when the December rankings were published. I had leapt 80 places to 29 in the world. I was only 5 places off the magic 24 which would remove the need for qualifying and make future tournaments that little bit easier. I had some more good news when I was granted a wild card entry into the British Open. This would be a great opportunity to test myself against the best, although I would have liked more time to prepare. The tournament was only a few weeks away so there was little I could do but rest. I was still determined not to overdo things.

The tournament was being held in Aberdeen. It was my first British Open for four years and it was great to be there competing. This was my third tournament, but the novelty still hadn't worn off. As soon as I arrived I spent as much time as possible sampling the atmosphere. It was good to see people like Jonah Barrington, who has become synonymous with the event. There were lots of others as well who I hadn't seen for years – people like Jonathan Power and Peter Nicol who had come to rule the roost since I had stopped playing. I chatted to both of them and they wished me well. My mum and dad came up to watch, which was nice. They hadn't seen me play since that ill-fated match against Jansher in the final four years earlier. I don't think they were too concerned with whether or not I won. They were just glad to see me back playing.

It was a great bonus not having to qualify, as it meant I would be fresh for the first round. The best players from all over the world were competing so I imagined I would probably come up against someone I had never played before. I couldn't have been more wrong. I was drawn against Alex Gough, a good friend who trained regularly with me in Nottingham. He would be a different proposition to most of the people I had played so far because he was in the top ten. I was nervous going into the match, but it worked out well for me and I won 3–1. Then I came up against David Evans who I had beaten five months earlier when I played in the World Cup for England against Wales. He was in good form, but I felt confident having beaten him once already.

I took the first game quite easily, then went ahead in the second but started to lose my way a little and he took it. It turned into a real battle, nip and tuck all the way with very little in it. I managed to take the third and hoped to gain control. To his credit, David came back and took the fourth. He proved a bit too strong for me and took the fifth. I was very disappointed to lose. Having won two tournaments, my hopes were high that I could do well in this one. It wasn't to be. I felt quite down about it because I felt I hadn't performed as well as I could have; if I don't perform to the top of my ability I get annoyed with myself.

Jonah Barrington came to speak to me and help me get things in perspective. His basic message was, what did I expect after being out of the game for so long? It takes time to get back to the very highest standard and to develop the consistency that goes with being a top player. I had done well but wasn't fully there yet. There were bound to be setbacks. He told me I had to give it more time. I knew he was right, but it wasn't necessarily what I wanted to hear so soon after the defeat. By the following day, I was starting to feel better about it. I had probably got a bit tired and didn't have the strength to continue playing at that pace. The strength would come. The good news was that physically I felt fine the next day.

As I looked back at the game, I realised that the main reason I had lost was that I'd simply been outplayed on the day. Yes, I got tired towards the end, but I couldn't use that as an excuse. If I had played better, I could have won it in three or four games and there would have been no need to go into a tiring fifth. My game wasn't quite strong enough, and my movement still left room for improvement. David was able to exploit that. While I was disappointed that I'd allowed him to do that, I took comfort in the fact that the defeat wasn't because my health had let me down. If that had been the case it would have been difficult to know what to do next. Faults in my game were much easier to tackle and I knew I would put them right over the following months.

Soon I began to feel more positive and took stock of my achievements. It was only nine months since I thought I would never play again. Yet in that time I had played in the World Cup, won my first two tournaments and reached the last 16 of the British Open. The defeat by David Evans was the first in my 17 games since returning from illness. Apart from that nervous qualifying match against Anthony Ricketts, it was the only time I had been taken to five games. I would have settled for that quite happily at the start of my comeback attempt.

Looking back, I realised it was probably a bit ambitious to expect to do well in such a major tournament so soon after returning. The British Open is a big event, with a big feel to it — it can be overpowering. The experience I gained there would stand me in good stead in the future. There was also the bonus that the win against Alex Gough should be enough to nudge me into the world's top 24 and remove the need to qualify for the big events. There was a lot to be pleased about and I started to feel a bit better although, try as I might, I couldn't help feeling disappointed at being outplayed.

I stayed on to enjoy the rest of the tournament and continue renewing old acquaintances. I kept a close eye on the other matches to see how people were playing. It might come in useful in the months to come. I was managing quite well in my mission to keep things in perspective and not get too concerned if things went wrong. By the end of the week, I was feeling very positive and really enjoying myself. I got roped into the exhibition doubles match that always precedes the singles finals. Doubles matches are always played for fun, and provide a little light relief before the tension of the main event. Jonah Barrington was the referee and got a great rapport going between the players and the crowd. At one point he brought the house down when he awarded a penalty point against me for playing a shot using only one hand. It was a nice touch in a nice event and I enjoyed myself immensely. I felt I now had a very good view of the bigger picture. It was looking better every day.

# 11.

## MIND GAMES

Most sports are now so physically demanding that it's easy to forget the crucial role psychology plays in determining success or failure. If you're not in the right frame of mind no amount of practice or fitness will save you. On the other hand, if you get things right mentally you're halfway there, even before you walk on court. Before I became ill, my mental strength was one of my main weapons. I don't think I was ever overawed by anyone or made to feel I couldn't win. It was quite the opposite; I nearly always fancied my chances, no matter who I was playing. When I returned after my illness, things were slightly different, of course. I still had great faith in my ability, but the uncertainty over my health obviously created some doubts.

These doubts persisted all the way through my first season back. As soon as I was asked to play for England, my first thoughts were to wonder whether I could still compete at that level. My three victories answered that question, but then there was the issue of whether or not I could compete over a whole tournament. Winning in Detroit and Pakistan proved that I could. There was one more major question to be answered, however. Was I good enough to go all the way back to the very top and challenge for the world number one slot?

My return put me in a situation that is probably unique in the history of the game. I was in my late twenties and a very experienced player. On the other hand, I had spent four years out and so in one sense I was like a newcomer to the scene. The new hierarchy which had emerged while I had been out were all people who were younger than I was, like Peter Nicol and Jonathan Power, now the masters of the game. Like any new challenger on the circuit, I regarded these players with great respect and saw them as the main people to beat if I was to re-establish myself at the

159

top. But there was also a part of me thinking of how I used to beat them on a regular basis before I became ill. How should I feel about playing them now? Should I be confident because I had always had the ascendancy over them in the past? Or should I be nervous, because this was now irrelevant and they had moved on to a higher standard that perhaps I could no longer reach? In truth, there were times when I wavered between the two extremes.

In all sports, you have to compete regularly against the best players if you want to reach their standard. It's a process that takes time. I realised that I might have to play and possibly lose several times to people like Nicol, Power and Simon Parke before I could reach the level I was once at and have a realistic chance of beating them. I also knew, however, that I would not be able to afford too many defeats if I were to turn the tables on them. The problem is that losing can become a habit after a while and makes you start to lose confidence.

Confidence is a fleeting thing. Once lost, it's very hard to get it back. If you lose to someone several times you can start thinking that he's better than you are. This feeling is hard to fight, no matter how many times you tell yourself it isn't true. It can create all sorts of mental blocks that make it difficult to reverse your defeats against the other player and start winning. You have to keep plugging away and hope to get a breakthrough. You would expect evenly matched players to share victories in an even fashion, win a few lose a few, but often it doesn't work out that way. It's not uncommon to see one player win six or seven times against the same opponent before he gets beaten. Then, when he does lose, he might suffer half a dozen defeats himself before he can regain the initiative.

You could argue that it's simply a case of one player being on better form than the other but I think there's more to it than that. If you win a few games against someone it gives you extra belief the next time you play them; if you lose a few, it puts all sorts of doubts in your mind. This was illustrated by the rivalry between Peter Nicol and Jonathan Power. At one point Power had a great run against Nicol, beating him nine times on the trot. Nicol was beating everyone else, even people who were beating Power at that time, but he couldn't reverse his string of defeats. You could see that Nicol was struggling mentally against Power. He lacked confidence and wasn't sure what to do. But, being the great player that he is, he kept plugging away. Then he made a breakthrough and got that all-important first victory. Perhaps he played better than usual that day; perhaps Power was below par. Whatever the reason, it prompted a complete reversal of fortune. Nicol went off on a series of victories himself, leaving Power to suffer the pangs of self-doubt. It was a complete reversal. In future matches, if Power lost the first game he found it hard to believe he could win.

It's strange how your mind plays tricks on you. I remember playing against Mark Cairns in a national league match when I was only 18 and very inexperienced at professional level. It was quite a close game, but then I got to match point. Mark is a very fine player and, naturally, he fought me all the way. He saved a few match points and we continued slugging it out. I wasn't too concerned. Then I reached match point again but, like the fighter he is, he managed to cling on again. I still didn't mind too much and was confident of winning, but by the time it had happened six times, I was starting to get a complex about it.

Up to that point, Mark had stayed in the game by his own efforts. Afterwards, however, I made it a lot easier for him because I started to doubt myself. My game deteriorated. I wasted a few more match points and started to wonder if I was ever going to find the winner. The more nervous I became, the more match points I threw away. It was becoming embarrassing. Then it got to a stage where I thought I just couldn't win, no matter what I did. I had no fewer than 14 match points that night, and couldn't convert any of them. Mark ended up taking it.

Thankfully, this was only a minor game and didn't blight me in any serious way. Other players have not been so lucky. Peter Nicol now has a great record in the British Open, but for several years he couldn't get past the first round. He was having great success in other big tournaments but somehow things always went wrong for him in the British. At first, it was probably just coincidence. He might have had the misfortune to come up against a good player, or perhaps he wasn't on top form once or twice. After these things happen four or five times, however, something in the back of your mind starts to make you doubt yourself. I think this was happening to Peter.

The changeover came about in a most unusual way. He was drawn against Paul Johnson in the 1997 tournament. Johnson had already lost to

Nicol a few times, and may have been starting to wonder if he would ever beat him. It was a good match and fortunately for Johnson, it went his way. Nicol lost when a stroke was called against him. He accepted the decision; the two players shook hands and walked off court. Johnson was delighted to have beaten Nicol in a major tournament and was no doubt looking forward to a long run of victories against him. It wasn't to be. His joy was short lived. The referee overturned the stroke decision against Nicol. The game wasn't over at all, and the two players had to go back on court.

You've probably guessed that Nicol went on to win. Not only that, but having overcome this mental block about getting beyond the first round, he then went all the way to the final, where it took Jansher Khan to stop him. He obviously got a taste for it because he was back the next year and, having done it once, he now had no trouble getting beyond the first round. In fact, he went all the way again and even avenged his defeat by Jansher the previous year by beating him and lifting the trophy. Not bad for a player who only 12 months earlier was wondering if he would ever get beyond the first round. Nicol's good fortune was bad news for Johnson, however. He was left wondering what on earth he had to do to beat Nicol. He thought he'd done it at last, only to have victory snatched away by the referee. He went on to suffer numerous defeats at the hands of Peter Nicol, sometimes after he had got himself into winning positions. There's little doubt the British Open game left psychological scars that took a long time to heal.

Problems of self-belief can emerge with players who've been part of squad coaching systems, which can sometimes lead to pecking orders that can be difficult for players to overcome. The player who starts as the best tends to remain the best and so on, down the line. This can persist even when lower-order players ought to be challenging for the top spot. Sometimes they don't succeed in doing so because they've got it into their heads that the player above them is better.

A lack of self-belief is apparent when youngsters start playing established pros. You can often tell from their body language and demeanour when they go on court that they don't believe they can win. And you can be certain that if someone thinks they're going to lose, then they almost certainly will. The problem can persist over several matches, over several years. You often see players competing against people they should be able to beat, but their mental block prevents it happening for them. Many young players seem to have preconceived notions about how well they can do. You can see them start well and match their opponent – they might take a game and everything looks good – but then they switch off mentally. It's almost as if they think they've got their token game and that's as much as they can hope for. They then seem to just go through the motions, waiting for the inevitable defeat to come. The better guy wins almost out of habit. It's what both players expect to happen, and it's like a self-fulfilling prophecy.

Often, watching a top-ranked player against someone lower down, you will find that there seems to be very little difference between them in the early stages of the game. It might be very tight and go to 13–13 and, on the face of it, there's nothing in it. Then the higher-ranked player goes on to win 15–13 and part of you thinks 'Well, it could have gone either way.' Deep down, though, you know that wasn't really the case. The better guy was never in any danger of losing it. He always had that little bit extra in reserve to call on when it mattered. It's partly ability, but it's also about belief. He's confident that when things get tight, he can play the better squash and that will carry him through.

People sometimes say: 'If that's the case, why doesn't the better player produce that form right at the start of the match? Why let the scores get so close before bringing out the extra quality?' There are various reasons for this. The top players sometimes need the extra mental stimulation of the big points at the end of a game to bring out the best in them. They're used to winning and are comfortable with it. When the tension mounts on the big points, they're confident they can stay calm and carry on playing well, while the lower-ranked player may freeze and see his game deteriorate. It's also partly because the lower-ranked player will be more psyched up at the start of a game. It's easier to motivate yourself to produce your best form when you're playing someone who is much better than you, than when you're playing someone who is much worse.

There's also a likelihood that the better player doesn't want to give it everything early on, especially if it's at the start of a tournament. When top athletes compete at the Olympic games, they don't try to break world records in the qualifying heats. They'll do whatever's necessary to get through and very little more because they want to save themselves for the final.

It's the same with top squash players. In the early rounds, they may be playing at 90 per cent of their ability whereas the lower-ranked player is going flat out. If the top player cuts it too fine and gets caught out in an early game, he will almost certainly go up a gear and quickly put things right in the next game. We saw this over and over again with Jansher. Sometimes his concentration seemed to waver in the early stages of a tournament and he would lose a game, perhaps 15–13 or 15–14. After that he would come back a different player and win the next few games very easily. He knew he could do this and, just as importantly, so did most of his opponents, which is why many of them would virtually give up after going one game ahead. They still couldn't bring themselves to believe they could win.

I was well aware of this psychological minefield from the time I started out as a professional at the age of 17. I got round it partly by setting myself different types of targets. Obviously players want to win every tournament right from the start, but I realised you had to be realistic. If you try to make yourself believe that you're going to win the world championship at your first attempt, then you risk losing confidence when you inevitably fail. It's far better to tailor your aims so that they're demanding enough to push you to the limit, but not so demanding that they create too much pressure.

I always gave 100 per cent but I realised that for a while I would have to measure my success in different ways than outright victory. If I was playing someone who I had a reasonable chance of beating, I would be disappointed with anything less than a win. On the other hand, if I was playing someone far better than me at that early stage then I accepted I would probably lose. That didn't mean, however, that I took things easy or had no targets – exactly the opposite. I would be looking to make the game as difficult as possible for my star opponent, even if he was almost certain to win in the end. I would fight him with everything I had on every single point. I would chase down every ball, run until I was ready to drop and then I would find yet more energy and come back at him for more. I wanted to see how well I could cope with the faster pace that comes with competing against better players, how well I could cover the court, dominate the T, get them out of position and trouble them with winning shots. Most likely they would win in the end, but they would certainly know they had been in a game.

When players are closely matched, confidence and inner belief is vital. How does a player develop these qualities? In lots of ways, but mainly through hard work and, just as important, by creating the right atmosphere and environment around him. The first thing is to make sure you get your preparation right. A lot of top sportsmen say that it's the background work they do before a tournament that gives them the confidence to cope with difficult situations. In training you work on all the tactics you will need. You practise against different types of players with a variety of styles. You develop your strengths, work on your weaknesses and try to recreate all the difficult situations you're likely to encounter in a game. The aim is to be so well honed that by the time you get to the tournament you hardly have to think about your game because it is all second nature. If you can get yourself this well prepared, then it establishes a deep core of self-belief and gives you the confidence to come through matches even though you might not be playing all that well on the day.

What constitutes the right preparation will vary from player to player. There is no right and wrong way. Each player has to do what works best for him or her. It's interesting to look at Nicol and Power again in this context. They might be two of the best around, but they have completely different personalities, contrasting styles, and opposing ideas on how the game should be approached. Nicol is in the traditional mould of the squash champion. He has great talent, of course, but his success depends on his determination, will to win and powers of concentration. You can be sure that his preparation will be meticulously thought out and followed through to the letter.

Power, on the other hand, doesn't have Nicol's powers of concentration and can lose his cool. His preparation is unlikely to be as thorough: it is quite likely that he would get bored with too many practice routines and too much physical training. On the other hand, he has far more flair and natural ability than Nicol. He may get downhearted if things are going badly, but when they are going well he can be unbelievably good. You see this in a lot of sports. People with a lot of flair often struggle with temperament, but they make up for it by being so creative. It makes them very exciting to watch because their inventiveness provides them with the weapons to be devastating on their day. Although they may not have the discipline to repeat the same form consistently, the times they do turn it on more than make up for that.

Flair players like Power and Brett Martin believe that too much practice can nullify players' inventiveness. In a way, they have a point. You often see players who are almost over-practised. They've worked their way through so many routines, like hitting the ball to the back of the court, that they've stopped thinking about what they're doing. Consequently, there's very little improvisation. It can make them worse players because they're so predictable and easy to read.

No one could say that about Martin or Power. If they were told to do set routines day in day out, they wouldn't be able to handle it mentally and it would probably have an adverse effect on their game. They're far better off going on court and practising in their own way. When you see them doing it, it sometimes looks as though they're just mucking about. They'll be playing different types of shots all the time and it may seem that there's no theory to it. But this unpredictable attitude is precisely what makes them difficult to play; you can never tell what they're about to do.

To make sure he's confident and relaxed for a big tournament, Nicol would pursue a disciplined regime, getting plenty of rest and looking after himself. He's unlikely to be having too many nights on the town. This is the way most coaches advocate that you should prepare for a big event. Some people, however, just aren't made to spend all their time playing and thinking about squash. Power is one of them. For him to impose a disciplined regime on himself would be counter-productive. Instead of feeling strong and relaxed, he would be bored and miserable. He would probably prefer to enjoy himself more, going out at night and generally having a good time. It wouldn't suit everyone and, in a way, perhaps he's lucky. He's one of those rare people who can do things naturally without too much training. Nicol would no doubt feel very nervous if he approached a tournament in this way. So would I, but it works for Power and that is the main point. Players must do whatever is best for them.

Both approaches carry their own dangers if taken too far. The relaxed approach can leave you ill-prepared physically, which may affect your confidence later if you feel you're not strong enough to compete. On the other hand, the more disciplined approach can leave you too mentally dependent on routine and everything being 'just right'. It can leave you vulnerable if something unexpected happens on the day of the big match. The tournament schedule might mean you can't practise at the time you think is best for your preparation; or perhaps you break your favourite racket or can't get the right food. I've always been pretty laid back about these things, but they can be minor catastrophes for anxious players who rely too much on perfect preparation. The player with the more relaxed approach will have the advantage in these circumstances because he's less likely to worry about changes in routine.

Many players now use sports psychologists to help them get in the right frame of mind. They're no substitute for good preparation, but they can certainly help you to relax and gain extra confidence. Psychologists encourage players to visualise the way they want to play before going on court, to see themselves going through the various aspects of their game. You might be on the T taking the ball quite early, hitting it tight into the back corner or playing a good drop shot. You imagine yourself moving smoothly around the court and visualise your opponent. You assess all his strengths and deal with them successfully. You go through all this and then when you go out on court, you feel as though you've been there already.

The psychologist can also help people deal with stress and worry, loss of concentration and controlling their temper. Players are taught to break down their fears and see them for what they really are pointless and irrelevant, for the main part. For example, someone might worry about having to travel the night before the game when really they want to rest. Maybe they are so nervous that they are unable to sleep. The reality is that these things will make very little difference. Most players have difficulty sleeping before a game, but once the action starts the adrenaline kicks in and everything is fine. Deep down players know this but sometimes they have to remind themselves of it. It's not the little problems that cause the damage it's the needless worry they create. The same thing applies to all sorts of imagined catastrophes and a session with the psychologist can help people see this.

An essential part of the right mental approach is having the will to win. Everyone wants to win, of course, but some people want it so badly that it becomes a formidable force. It's definitely been prominent in all the great champions from the days of Jonah Barrington and Geoff Hunt, through to the mighty Khans and now the modern day with the likes of Peter Nicol. Unlike a lot of other mental qualities, it can't really be developed. It's either a part of your make-up or it isn't. The will to win is one of Nicol's most formidable qualities. It enables him to win matches from positions that would cause other players to throw in the towel. He's had situations where he's been down in games and looked certain to be defeated, where he's on his last legs, but somehow he gets some energy from somewhere, makes a big push and comes back to win.

Simon Parke is the same. He will give it everything right up to the last rally, no matter how exhausted he feels. This can put enormous pressure on people. If you know you're up against a player who will never give in it creates doubts in your mind. You never feel comfortable because you know they're likely to come back at you no matter how far ahead you get. It can make you tense and affect your game as you wait in dread for the fightback. Some players can feel intimidated and not want to carry on because they know the other will force them through the pain barrier. The ability to push yourself is a crucial thing in squash, and often separates the champions from the also-rans.

The crowd can also have a huge bearing on a match. Many of our top events are held in Egypt now, and they're always lively and colourful affairs. The organisers do everything they can to make foreign players welcome but they can't do much about the fervour of the fans. The crowds get behind the local players and are very raucous in their support. They not only cheer on their own favourite but can also be quite hostile to the opponent, often cheering any mistakes he makes. It can be an intimidating atmosphere and players have to be strong to cope with it. So do the referees. They come from all over the world and there's no question of them being biased in favour of the home players, but nevertheless it must sometimes be difficult for them not to feel slightly influenced when called upon to decide on borderline calls for lets and strokes.

I think this pressure got to Rodney Eyles when he played the Egyptian star Ahmed Barada in the final of the Al Ahram tournament in 1996.

Barada is a very fine player but Eyles was a seasoned campaigner and most people would have expected him to win. At least, they would have if the game had not been held in Egypt. Eyles is an aggressive player who wears his heart on his sleeve. The hostile crowd and questionable refereeing decisions may have had an effect on his game. He lost when many people thought he ought to have won.

It would be wrong to imagine that the crowd would always swing things in favour of the home star. The support can be a great help, but it also brings its own problems because it can be hard to live up to the level of expectation. Everyone wants you to win and you don't want to let people down. This pressure might not be too bad if you're winning easily, but it can make players tense if the match gets very close. For instance, it may have been a significant factor when Peter Nicol played Barada in the Al Ahram tournament in 1999. As we have seen, Nicol is very strong mentally and was able to withstand the pressures of the crowd. He kept the game close and this threw the pressure back on to Barada, who was aware that people would be disappointed if he didn't pull off the expected win. It may well have got to him and he ended up losing.

If you get your preparation right and everything goes well for you then you might make it through to the final. But even then, there's no way of knowing how you're going to feel on the big day. People who have been to numerous finals will tell you there's no set pattern to how they will react. It can be different with every match. No matter how rigid the preparation, players are not machines: they may feel up or down for no other reason than the vagaries of human nature and the normal everyday changes in mood. I don't think anyone could claim that they've felt excited and positive about every game they've played. All you can do is be aware of your feelings and try to deal with them. If you're feeling very positive and confident, you may have to remind yourself to remain on your guard and not become too complacent. If for some reason you feel a little down or negative, on the other hand, you have to build yourself up and think positively about how you can win the match.

Whatever your mood, you will inevitably feel pumped up. It's important to find ways to relax; you have to find some kind of equilibrium between feeling determined yet calm. You have to want to win, yet you mustn't put yourself under so much pressure that you won't be able to perform. It's a delicate balancing act in which players will draw on all their experience. They'll remember all the preparation they've done, remind themselves of what the psychologists have told them or perhaps go through their own routines for getting in the right frame of mind. Players who've been in big finals before have a tremendous advantage because they can avoid any past mistakes and repeat the things they've got right. The newcomer has it all to learn.

Some people like to shut themselves off from everyone before a match. I remember seeing Chris Dittmar on the day he played Jansher Khan in the final of the British Open. He was totally focused and didn't want to speak to anyone. Other people do the opposite and like to chat, anything but think about the match. I tend to spend about half an hour early in the day working out how I'm going to play and then I just want to put it out of my mind. I try to surround myself with familiar things, perhaps listen to my favourite music or relax with friends. But no matter what you do, your pre-tournament preparation hardly ever goes exactly as you plan. Again, the important thing is not to let it get to you.

Once players are at the top level and constantly reaching the finals and semi-finals of the big tournaments, there's often very little to distinguish them in terms of ability and commitment. Winning and losing can come down to how well they perform on a few big points. Finals will often start a bit tentatively as players test each other out. Towards the middle of the match, they will both be well into their stride and probably playing their best-quality squash. As things reach a climax, however, the standard is likely to drop again because each player is probably getting nervous. The drop in standard in purist terms is more than made up for by the increase in excitement.

Then comes decision time; match ball in the deciding frame. This is where players have to dig deep and summon up every ounce of self-belief. It's not really a question of ability at this stage. It's who can hold themselves together better. At 14–14 it's all too easy to tense up. The same applies if you're serving to win the match or struggling to stay in it: you're likely to be just as nervous whatever the case. You're frightened of making a mistake, but you also know that if you start playing tentatively you may start to lose.

In the past, when things got tight or if a player was doing badly and falling behind, he might try to steady his game and work his way back into the match. The idea was to be cautious and not make any silly mistakes. This had certain advantages, in the sense that you were less likely to give much away. On the other hand, it would make your game predictable and unthreatening. It also meant you might be conditioned not to go for winning shots even when the opportunity arose. Nowadays, many players will go to the opposite extreme – all-out attack. You will often see the game finely poised at 14–14. Both players will be very anxious; a bit of gamesmanship might be coming into it; more lets might be called than earlier in the game; there might be a suspicion that the players are getting in each other's way a little. These are nerve-racking times, and exactly the moments when players would have opted for caution in the past. Some will do so even now but you're also just as likely to see a willingness to suddenly go for winning shots.

The server might hit a slightly loose ball. Nine times out of ten, the opponent would hit tight down the wall to the back but might suddenly throw caution to the wind and drop it short at the front, hoping to find the nick and win the game. It's very risky but people are prepared to go for it more and more, with the theory that the attacking player will win more often than not. A similar approach is often seen when someone who isn't playing very well falls a long way behind. If a player looks like losing, the conventional wisdom of the past is that people should try to steady things down and work their way back into the match. Instead, people sometimes go for winning shots from unexpected places. It's a risky tactic, but it can work because it's the last thing the opponent expects.

In squash, perhaps more than in most other sports, it's the unusual that catches you out. I've seen it work several times, once against me, unfortunately, when I played Chris Dittmar in the Leekes Welsh classic. It was 2–2. I was well ahead in the fifth game and looked set to win. I expected Dittmar to dig deep and try to grind his way back into the game. Instead, he totally surprised me by rattling off six outright winners in the space of a few moments and took the match. They were all very risky shots and could just as easily have lost him the game, but on that occasion it worked.

Jansher Khan did something similar against Simon Parke in the World Open in Cyprus in 1995. In one of the games, Simon was 13–6 up and looked to be coasting. Then Jansher hit nine outright winners and took the game before Simon knew what was happening. Peter Nicol took the same approach against Martin Heath in the World Open in 1999. Heath was 12–8 up and controlling the match. Everyone expected a cautious player like Nicol to try to steady the game down. Instead, he went on an attacking spree and hit five or six winners one after another. It worked and he took the game.

The element of surprise is vital in this, of course. It probably wouldn't work if players did it all the time, but used sparingly it can catch people out. In a way it's not as brave as it might seem; if you've fallen behind it's probably because your tactics up to that point haven't been working. The chances are that if you stick to the same routine, or play even more cautiously, then you'll probably lose anyway. However, if you suddenly attack you may shake off whatever has been holding you back and take the opponent by surprise. You may just snatch victory when all seemed lost.

Squash players are learning more about how to prepare and get the best out of themselves, but it's still difficult to pull it all together at the same time. When players do feel they've got everything right, both mentally and physically, they talk about being 'in the zone'. This simply means they're in peak condition and playing as well as they possibly can. Some people say that when they've won a match in these conditions they've played almost as though they were on autopilot: everything just clicked. It's not that common, but it's great when it happens. You can play like someone possessed and pull off some of the best victories of your life.

A great example was the performance of Rodney Eyles against Peter Nicol in the final of the World Championships in Malaysia in 1997. Eyles had been around a long time without winning many big titles. Nicol was very much the rising star at that time, in the process of eclipsing the fading Jansher Khan. Most people expected Nicol to win. They hadn't reckoned on Eyles playing the best squash of his life. He had one of those perfect matches that perhaps only happen once or twice in a career. He was brilliant; physically strong, mentally resilient and totally focused. Nicol showed all the qualities we've come to associate with him but he couldn't do a thing about it. Eyles was unstoppable. All squash players would love to be able to find that kind of form on a regular basis but, sadly, it's the exception rather than the rule.

I've experienced most of the tricks that the mind can play on a professional player and have dealt with most of them. In a way, perhaps I'm lucky. I've never feared anyone and I always feel I can win. On the other hand, I also know that confidence doesn't come out of thin air. It has to be earned by preparing properly and that's something I've always tried to do. Players' needs change over the years, however. Since returning to the circuit, the main challenge has been to make sure I remain relaxed — easier said than done in professional sport.

I still want to win the British Open or the world championship and get to world number one. After my lay-off, I'm probably one of the hungriest players on the circuit, but I'm determined to keep things in perspective. If I ever feel down because things aren't going as well as I would like, I remind myself of all those years when I was out of the game and couldn't play at all.

# 12.

## A KINDER WAY TO FITNESS

The years when I was forced out of the game by CFS revolutionised my thinking about fitness and methods of training. Throughout that time, I was always worried that I would fall so far behind the top players that I would never be able to get back on level terms. Then, when I did finally make it back, I was amazed that I picked up fitness so quickly. I realised that if you work hard when you're young, you build up a good foundation that stays with you even when you ease off. I came to see that a lot of the training I had done in the past might have been unnecessary. You have to go through a period of working very hard but if you go too far, it can be a waste of time. You can overtrain.

I had worked ferociously hard when I was younger. Probably I did too much and damaged my health. Ironically, in doing so I still managed to build up a base level of fitness that enabled me to start playing again remarkably quickly. I knew that my training routines would have to be different if I were to get the best out of myself in the future. The trick was to make sure I did enough work to be fit but not so much that I became too tired. This can be a difficult balance to achieve. I was brought up in the hard school of training, pioneered by Jonah Barrington and later developed by Geoff Hunt and Jahingir Khan.

Jonah Barrington was the first person to start taking squash training seriously. Before him, squash was an amateurish game with an amateurish approach to fitness. Training was little more than a bit of running and the occasional press-up. In fact, many players at that time considered training somewhat ungentlemanly and against the spirit of the game. Jonah changed all that. He set about creating training routines that were not only punishing but also specially designed for squash. He invented ghosting, which involves moving around the court going through the motions of playing a shot but without a ball or racket. It looks a bit odd but it works. The idea is to increase your fitness at the same time as improving your technique and positioning.

Jonah's dedication to fitness is now legendary. He pushed himself to the limit and beyond. In fact, he still trains as hard as Simon Parke, as I found out when Simon and I went to stay with him a few years ago. He mapped out a squash court on his lawn and had us doing exercises like ghosting and shuttle runs. I remember his children, who are enthusiastic players but not as keen as he is, looking at us in disbelief. They thought we were mad. I can't imagine that any sportsman ever worked harder than Jonah did. Today's squash players certainly don't, and that is in no way a criticism of them. The fact is that Jonah, by his own admission, probably overdid things with his monk-like lifestyle and fanatical dedication to physical fitness. He once described himself as the human guinea pig because he had tested out so many new techniques. Some were very successful, and are still used by squash players today. Others were less helpful and ended up causing Jonah physical damage. We all owe him a great deal. He led the way and, by trial and error, discovered what was useful and what wasn't.

Geoff Hunt was also totally dedicated, especially after Jonah Barrington upped the stakes with his levels of fitness. Hunt would often train doing 400-metre sprints, taking a 45-second rest between each one. He might repeat the routine up to 30 times. That seems over the top now; most players wouldn't do more than 10 or 15 repetitions. The legacy of Hunt and Barrington was taken up by Jahingir Khan. He often followed up gruelling on-court training sessions with ten-mile runs through the mountains of his native Pakistan.

The principles of hard training were instilled into me at an early age. I remember going to training camps with the England squad when I was 11 or 12. We were only children, yet we were put through gruelling sessions doing everything from court sprints to throwing medicine balls to each other. We would come back home feeling totally exhausted. Our trainers were well-meaning and only following the best advice of the time, but I don't think many experts today would want to work children so hard. It was a similar attitude years later when we trained with the England Under-23 squads. These sessions might last three days and we would come back feeling shattered. Most of us wouldn't do anything for several days afterwards, which seemed to defeat the object of having worked so hard in the first place.

With this sort of background, it's perhaps not surprising that I put such a premium on fitness when I was younger. The fact that I was so driven to succeed, and so determined to overtake Jansher Khan at the top, meant there was always a danger that I would overdo things. I didn't realise it at the time, but I see now that I did train too hard during my late teens and early 20s. I would think nothing of doing a gruelling session in the morning followed by a hard training game in the afternoon and perhaps some gym work in the evening. I very rarely gave myself enough time to recover. If I felt tired, I was more likely to think that I needed to train harder than to consider that perhaps I needed to take things easier.

Now I realise that this approach was often counter-productive, and even cost me some matches. I remember losing to Tristan Nancarrow in the second round of the British Open in 1992. He was a good player and I don't want to make excuses; I might have lost anyway. But there's no doubt in my mind that I had tired myself out by working too hard before the tournament. I had played hard practice games the day before my first match. That was quite common in those days. Many great players like Ross Norman said they didn't feel right unless they had some tough sessions immediately before the tournament. It was very much the accepted wisdom, but it sometimes meant I was already tired before the event even started. It was the wrong approach, but I was probably able to get away with it in those days because I was so young and strong. There's no way I could do so now.

My new approach to training makes the need for rest just as important as the need to work hard. If I'm in any doubt, I will rest rather than train. Exactly how much training I do depends on the time of year. During the season when the tournaments are coming in quick succession, I don't do very much at all. Most players don't. In the week immediately before a big event, I try to get as much rest as possible. I might play the odd practice game and spend a bit of time on court working on technique, but little else. The main objective at this point is to arrive at the tournament feeling fresh. This enforced relaxation can be difficult to come to terms with mentally, because it's easy to feel you might lose some speed or sharpness.

However, I've learnt from experience that that doesn't happen nearly as much as you imagine. If you've got your basic fitness laid down and you prepare properly, then you won't lose much by resting.

It's significant that many top players are now coming to this conclusion. I remember talking to Peter Nicol a few years after I became ill and he told me that he had cut down on the amount of training he did. This was surprising at the time because he too was in the long tradition of squash players who worked themselves to the limit. He told me he had decided to ease back, partly because of what happened to me but also because he was coming to see that it wasn't necessary to train so hard. It was obviously a risk, but it has certainly worked for him over the last few years.

The body needs time to recover after a hard match or training session. If you push yourself on to further efforts without getting enough rest you will do yourself more harm than good. Not only because you risk tiring yourself or damaging your body, but also in terms of your attitude to the game. It's as important to be as keen as possible before a match as it is to be fit, and it's hard to be enthusiastic if you're physically and mentally jaded from too much work. You're likely to find all your effort has been counter-productive and you simply don't have the energy or the appetite to play well. That's what happened to me against Nancarrow.

Players are now urged to rest more and give themselves days off during the week so their bodies can recover. These recovery periods can be active or passive. Passive recovery is very straightforward, and simply means resting totally; active recovery could involve gentle winding-down exercises such as an easy session on a bike. Some people feel it's often better to do something simple than do nothing at all. Massages are another form of active recovery. They're very relaxing and help to ease away tension in the muscles.

As with all players, most of my serious training is done in the summer before the season starts. This is where you create the bedrock of fitness that will see you through the rest of the year. If you do it properly, you'll only have to keep playing and doing the odd session to keep things topped up. If you don't get it right, it's unlikely that you'll be able to catch up during the season. There isn't time to do much training once the tournaments get under way.

I have a two-month training programme drawn up with the help of sports scientists, designed to lead me up to the start of the season. I like to fit in a number of different types of exercise every week. These include gym sessions, hill running, court sprints, ghosting and so on. I do them in a certain order. For example, if I wanted to do a hard session in the gym then I would probably do it first thing in the morning to get the most out of it. If I played a match first, I might feel a bit tired and not be able to put as much effort into the weights as I would like. Although it's all written down the programme is very flexible, and I often change things round. If I'm feeling tired I might ease off, but on the other hand, if things are going very well then I might do more. A lot depends on whether people are around to play against. I might have a training session planned for the afternoon, but if a top player like Simon Parke or Martin Heath is around I'll take the opportunity to play a match instead. Conversely, if you have a match planned but your opponent can't make it, it's back to the training routines.

The programme takes account of my illness. If I do too much endurance work I can start to feel tired, so I make sure not to overdo things. I'm lucky in one respect because my endurance is generally good anyway, without needing too much work. Players vary a great deal in this respect. Some have to work hard at stamina, but I don't. However, I have to concentrate more on speed and power because those things don't come so easily to me. The new regime is much gentler than the training schedules I followed in the past. Before I became ill, I would train hard nearly every day. Looking back, it was probably too intense and didn't allow enough time for recovery.

A hard day now might see me getting up at about 8.30 a.m. and going on court to do some racket work for about 75 minutes. This isn't particularly tiring because it's all about practising shots and perfecting technique. While I'm working, I make sure I drink plenty of water. I also like to use carbohydrate drinks which help keep energy levels up. After the skills work, I might do 75 minutes in the gym lifting weights. That would take me up to lunchtime. I would then rest, or maybe go back to bed for an hour. In the afternoon I might play a hard practice match and follow that up with a long session stretching out. That would probably be it for the day. If I were going to have an evening session, say a practice match against a top player, then I would probably do very little in the afternoon. Instead, I would make sure I got plenty of rest. If I start to feel unwell then I'm quite prepared to take a day or two off. In the past I would have felt guilty about that and worry that I would lose out. I'm a lot more relaxed now.

I have to accept that the CFS, or my proneness to CFS, is still there. It's very important not to do anything to trigger it off again. So far, I seem to be managing quite well but there are still times when I don't feel 100 per cent; I'm not even sure what 100 per cent is for me any more. Maybe I'm not capable of being as good as I once was. I have to accept my limitations. Nowadays, I realise that not every training session has to be flat out. I can vary things and perhaps only give 80 per cent at times. Heart monitors help in this respect by enabling me to work within certain levels.

Although the training routines I use now are much less demanding than when I first started out, they're not that different from the approach taken by most modern players. There's been a wind of change since the days of Barrington, Hunt and Jahingir Khan. Those three greats won 24 British Open titles among them, so it's hard to argue with their methods. The fact is, though, that they were training for a different type of game to the one played today. The players of the '80s and early '90s used heavy wooden rackets which made it hard to get any real power on the ball. They played on warm, solid wall courts that gave the ball plenty of bounce and made it more difficult to kill. The tin was two inches higher, which again made it more difficult to play a winning shot.

Those factors taken together meant the rallies tended to go on for several minutes because it was so difficult for anyone to put the ball away. Big matches tended to be exhausting wars of attrition lasting well over two hours. I've watched videos of matches between players like Barrington and Hunt. The percentage of shots hit to the back wall was much higher than it is now. They didn't have to get to the front of the court as much as players do today. There was less need for speed and quick reactions, but there was probably more need for stamina. The winner in those days was often the one who was best able to last the pace. Small wonder, then, that the stars of that era put so much emphasis on endurance.

The modern glass courts, lighter rackets and the lower tin mean that the game is now faster and more attacking. The rallies don't tend to last as long, but probably contain a greater variety of shots. The changes may seem subtle, but they're vitally important because they call for a different type of fitness. Thankfully, unlike Jonah Barrington, players today don't have to rely on trial and error to find the right way to train. They can call on an army of experts to guide them. This was one of the things that developed during the years I was out of the game. When I started out players were left to their own devices, as they were in Jonah's day. Now, because of lottery funding, we have a lot of help from sports scientists, psychologists and nutritionists. It's a massive leap forward.

Endurance training is still needed because squash is one of the toughest sports around. Even now big games can last a long time, and you have to play at least five matches in five days to win a major tournament. Players still do a lot of stamina work, but have to be fast to get to the front of the court, because the ball dies so quickly. Players have therefore adapted their training to the requirements of the modern game: it calls for strength, speed, agility and flexibility as much as endurance. You need to get all of these areas right to prepare properly for the way the game is played today.

We do a lot more work in the gym now than when I first started out. This is mainly to build overall strength, particularly in the legs, to increase your speed on court. It's important to develop the stomach muscles as well because, surprisingly perhaps, they also play a part in enabling you to move faster. We also do upper body exercises for overall strength and stability, but this is not as important as the other areas. In all the gym work, you have to be careful to use only medium weights. Too much work with heavier weights would start to make you bigger and slower, which would defeat the object. The idea is to be strong but lean, rather than big and bulky.

Mobility is also very important, so I use routines putting cones close together on court and then running in between them. I also spend a lot of time on plymetrics, which involves things like skipping, hopping and bounding. All these exercises develop your leg muscles to give you extra spring from the floor. This is very important in a game that involves racing in constantly changing directions in order to retrieve the ball, and then having to push back to be in position for the next shot. Some players also do lunges to give them extra spring. Another good exercise for developing strength and good footwork is to place a ladder on court and then step in and out of the different sections. You can move forwards, sideways or backwards.

Ghosting is still very popular because it gives you speed, mobility and endurance all in one. Some players do the exercises carrying weights so they get even stronger. The movement then seems a lot easier once they take the weights off for a game. Again, the emphasis is on short bursts rather than long endurance work. You might do ghosting for a minute, then rest for 30 seconds. The idea is to repeat this about ten times. In the past, players might have spent over two minutes ghosting before they rested. That would help with endurance but wouldn't be as good for speed. I also like to do a lot of work on the bike. It builds up strength in the legs but doesn't cause too much wear and tear on the joints. This is important, because the constant twisting and turning on court can cause enough problems without adding to them with your training.

Playing practice matches is one of the best and most enjoyable forms of training. You wouldn't go far wrong if you just played hard matches every day. In fact, ghosting and playing practice matches now accounts for about 80 per cent of my physical training. However, I still feel it's necessary to do some running and gym work to make sure all my muscles are being developed properly. Playing on its own will develop some muscles more than others. This can cause imbalances which could lead to injuries. Gym work evens out these imbalances and so reduces the risk of injury.

Most of today's top players spend less time training than the stars of the past. The emphasis now is on quality rather than quantity. You won't gain a great deal from training for hours on end, day in day out. Most players don't enjoy training. Ghosting or running round cones aren't the kind of things people do for fun, and hardly anyone carries on with them once they've stopped playing professionally. It's therefore important to recognise the things you like doing and concentrate on them. It's best to avoid things you don't enjoy. If you hate hill running, then there's no point in incorporating too much of it into your training programme, because it will only bring you down and possibly demotivate you. There's no fixed or correct routine. It's very much a personal thing. Different training methods suit different people and you have to find what suits you.

The change in approach to training is reflected in the way fitness is now assessed by the sports scientists. They used to measure our progress by making us run on the treadmill. Now, they have a machine that measures how quickly you can perform ghosting routines. It bleeps intermittently and you have to run from the T to the corner of the court in between each bleep. The coaches can increase the speed of the bleeps until you reach your limit. Then you have a benchmark by which to measure your progress. It's a simple thing, but it's a big advance on what we had before, because it's specific to squash. Running on a treadmill is good for general fitness, but it doesn't reproduce the conditions of playing a match. All it really qualifies you for is more running on a treadmill, which is of little use. In fact, it may even make you slower because it diverts your attention away from work that will increase your speed.

Most players today place a lot of emphasis on flexibility and the need to stretch before and after a hard session. The value of stretching was drilled into us when we were younger, but we didn't always bother. Now that has all changed because people realise the importance of being supple, especially in a game like squash which is very severe. Muscles can get very tight when they've been forced to work hard, and that can make them prone to injuries. Stretching helps them recover and reduces the risk. A lot of players will stretch for at least 20 minutes before and immediately after a match. When they're training, they might spend up to 40 minutes doing nothing but stretching. Flexibility is so important in a game where you are constantly turning and changing direction.

Diet is probably given a lot more emphasis than it was in the past. The nutritionists advise plenty of carbohydrates like bread, pasta and potatoes. They also recommend meat and other protein sources to help in repairing damaged muscles. Some players take nutrition very seriously, but others don't worry too much about it. They argue that there's no point in eating all the right foods if you don't enjoy them. It will only make you miserable and consequently have a detrimental effect on your game. For them, it's far better to eat what they like and what keeps them happy. At least they're not likely to put on too much weight, because they burn up so much energy.

There's also a much more relaxed attitude towards players enjoying themselves off court. Years ago it was considered that if you went out for a few beers, it would badly affect your game. Now the consensus is that if you drink in moderation it probably won't hurt you – it's the same argument that applies to food. It's not in some players' characters to live a life of total abstinence. They would become miserable and might even use it as an excuse to themselves not to play well. The lifestyle of doing nothing but training and preparing for squash has completely gone. It's not necessary to go over the top. People feel they need to enjoy life in order to get the best out of themselves.

Exactly how much enjoyment is needed will, of course, vary from player to player. But no matter who you are, you have to keep things to moderate levels. Getting drunk three times a week will very quickly show itself in your form. I have a few beers once or twice a week and perhaps a more generous session once a month or so. It's down to the individual. Some people can let their hair down every week without any adverse effect. I certainly can't do that. Perhaps it's the CFS, but I don't seem to have as much alcohol tolerance as many other people so I have to be that bit more careful. I need to be able to make the most of the time I have left playing squash. Nevertheless, I think it's important to relax and enjoy a few drinks with friends.

No matter how hard you train, the most important thing is to be able to play. Most of your time should be taken up practising shots and grooving techniques. This may sound like stating the obvious but there is still a feeling among some people that squash is all about stamina. This may be a hangover from the days of Jonah Barrington; a mythology has grown up around him and his amazing levels of fitness. It's true that he worked hard, but that perhaps overshadows the fact that he was also a very skilful player who spent hours practising his skills. He knows as much about technique as anyone. People sometimes forget that because so much attention has been paid to his fitness. I still speak to him on a regular basis, and our conversations are as much about the finer points of how the game should be played as they are about training methods.

That's how it should be: squash is essentially a game of skill. It was Jonah's skill as much as his fitness that enabled him to be such a great champion. It's likely that in future, skill will be at an even greater premium and players will have to come to terms with that or be left behind.

# 13

# BRITISH CHAMPION AGAIN

Squash doesn't have permanent homes in the way that English football and tennis have Wembley and Wimbledon. This means courts and seating have to be specially constructed for big tournaments, leading to some wonderful and occasionally bizarre surroundings. In Egypt, for example, where everyone is squash mad, they stage their national Al Ahram tournament in the open air, right next to the Pyramids. This creates a sense of the surreal, especially at night when the gloom of the ancient monuments is bathed in floodlighting from the courts and the arena. The peace of the resting pharaohs is constantly disturbed by the modern-day Egyptians cheering on their local heroes. It all seems incongruous, but somehow it works and creates a wonderful atmosphere. It's a measure of the sport's popularity that it's allowed to disturb the peace in this way. No other event is allowed anywhere near the monuments.

The Americans have nothing like the Pyramids, but they have Grand Central Station in New York. For the Tournament of Champions, they construct a big arena in the open concourse area. Again, it's a little unusual but it works, not only providing a great venue but bringing the game to the attention of millions of commuters as they pass through the station every day. Squash is becoming more popular across the Atlantic, and the United States now provides some of the sport's best events.

The Tournament of Champions in February 2000 was the next big tournament after my appearance in the British Open, when I lost to David Evans. There was a gap of six weeks so I had plenty of time to prepare and assess my progress. That was just as well, as I had a bit of a scare immediately after the British Open. I went home for Christmas to relax and look forward with everyone else to the millennium celebrations. I got flu. I didn't want to get too concerned, but I wondered if this was a sign that the CFS was coming back. I needn't have worried. Just about everyone seemed to get flu that year. The newspapers and TV were full of stories about how the health service couldn't cope.

I quickly recovered and started looking forward to going to America. I was also considering whether to play in the British National championships which followed a week after the New York tournament. I wanted to play in both, but wasn't sure how I would cope with two events in such quick succession. The organisers wanted me to decide but I didn't feel I could make a commitment. I didn't want to let anyone down if I couldn't make it, and neither did I want to feel pressurised into playing if I didn't feel fully fit. I decided to wait until I came back from America before I made up my mind.

The six-week gap before I had to fly to America gave me my first chance to do some real training since the previous summer. I devised a programme to see how I would cope. I worked hard over the following weeks, and was delighted to find that I came through it all right. I could feel myself getting stronger and stronger. Other people might take this for granted when they do a lot of training, but I couldn't. Over the previous four years, training would sometimes make me feel weaker and more tired. It was a great boost to me.

The training continued to go well, however, and I set off for New York feeling strong and confident. The Big Apple is a favourite venue for many players, for obvious reasons. The place is bursting with life and there's so much to do there. Playing a tournament is hardly a holiday but I was determined to enjoy myself while I was there and at least see some of the city. I flew out about a week early with Simon Parke and a few others. We visited a few of the main sights like Times Square, Central Park and Soho. We also took in a few good restaurants, but the spectre of the tournament loomed large and dominated our thinking. You can't relax much no matter how enticing the surroundings, because your mind always returns to the job in hand and the need to prepare properly. We still had to practise and get plenty of rest. That meant walking around the city had to be limited. Even something so seemingly innocent as sightseeing can be tiring when you're trying to get the maximum out of yourself.

I was now ranked 19 in the world, so I didn't have to play in the qualifying rounds. That was a great help and meant I would be fresh for my first-round match against Thierry Lincou, my opponent in the semi-final of the Pakistan Open. It turned out to be a very similar game; a hard physical battle. I won 3–2 but wasn't happy with the way I had played; not as sharp or accurate as I wanted to be. In the next round, I played Paul Johnson. He was ranked 6 in the world and it was a big step up. I felt I was back with the big boys now. It turned out to be a massive struggle. The increase in standard was quite apparent as soon as Paul came out. He's a great player, and he started at a very fast pace. Paul played tremendously and although the games were close, he took a 2–0 lead. I had to win the remaining games to stay in the tournament. The good thing from my point of view was that although it had been a very tough match, I still felt strong.

I managed to hang in there and gradually started to turn it round. It was close all the way but I took the next two games to level it. The irony was that Paul was probably the one who started to tire first. Recently in tournaments it had been the other way round, with me getting weaker while the other player grew stronger. It was a welcome role reversal as far as I was concerned. The match lasted well over two hours and went on past midnight. I got more into it as the game went on and started to play better. Paul may have taken too much out of himself in the first two games and I finished the stronger, taking it in the fifth. I was delighted because I had beaten the world number six, but I also took great satisfaction from the fact that I had felt so strong and kept going to the end.

The next day brought an even bigger challenge; the world number one, Peter Nicol. I had beaten Nicol several times before I became ill, but this was now a different game altogether. He had obviously improved, whereas I had gone the other way because of my illness. I had made great strides in the last six months, but was it enough to cope with the best player in the world? It would be an interesting test and I was really looking forward to it.

Nicol went into the game as a definite favourite, not only because of his position in the rankings but also because he was probably fresher than I was. He had got through the first two rounds with comfortable 3–0 victories whereas I had faced two hard five-set matches. I didn't see that as any reason to make excuses. It was up to me to get in a similar position by playing better and securing 3–0 victories myself. That's the way great champions win tournaments. They get through the early rounds easily and save their energy for the tougher matches that follow.

Any question marks in my mind about the difference in standard between us were answered within minutes of going on court. Nicol came out like a train from Grand Central Station. I didn't know what had hit me and by the time I'd settled down, I had lost the first game 15–4. Afterwards, some fans and reporters put my poor start down to the fact that I was still stiff from the marathon matches on the two previous days. This was partly true, but the main reason was simply my difficulty coping with the quality of his play. As world champion, he was that bit sharper than anyone else I had come up against since my return. He was a level higher, taking the ball that fraction earlier and putting it away into the corners. I wasn't used to that kind of pace and accuracy. You can't get used to it until you play against it. In that sense, coming up against Nicol was another stepping stone towards my rehabilitation at the top level.

It was interesting to play him and see how his game had improved while I had been out. Nicol had always been a steady player who was very effective without ever looking that dynamic. He didn't hit the ball very hard but played it to a good length, which made it difficult for his opponent to attack. He never made you feel under any great pressure, as if he were going to blitz you off court or hit lots of clever winners. He volleyed a great deal and was good around the middle of the court. One of his greatest assets was his tremendous mental strength.

The first thing I noticed when we started playing was that his short game was much better, although he still wasn't that clinical in putting the ball away. He had more control and his movement was more economical. Overall, he was a better player than when I had last played him and it wasn't surprising that he was the world number one. He had no significant weakness although there were a few chinks I could exploit; like a lot of left-handers, he was a bit more vulnerable in his backhand corner. For a player of his standard, he struggled a bit when you paused a little before playing your shot, forcing him to check his stride before moving off again. They were only relative weaknesses, of course, but I tried to make the most of them.

Thankfully, I was able to recover after my drubbing of the first game and adjust to the higher standard. I won the second game quite comfortably and then took a 14–11 lead in the third. At that point, I thought I had a good chance of winning but he came back with three good points to level the game. I was then left to decide whether to play to 15 or 17 points. Fifteen would make it a game of sudden death, with the next point being the winner. Seventeen would prolong the game and give me the cushion of a few points to settle down and get back into my stride. To some people's surprise, I chose 15. The next point would be the winner. Unfortunately for me, I lost it and went 2–1 down.

Afterwards, some people asked why I chose the sudden death option and wondered if it was because I was tired and wanted to avoid having to play any more points than were necessary. It was true that I was starting to feel a little tired, but that had nothing to do with my decision. I was working on the simple law of averages. The game had been nip and tuck all the way with never more than a few points in it. Then suddenly Nicol took three points in a row. Given the way the game had gone up to then, the likelihood was that the next point would go to me. It didn't work out that way but the theory was sound and I would make the same decision again.

Nevertheless, it was a big blow to lose that game. At 2–1 up, I would have fancied my chances. At 2–1 down it was going to be very difficult. And so it turned out. I faded in the fourth game and he took it quite easily. I was feeling a bit tired, partly from the two previous matches but also because this game had been so tough. It was a real step up in standard and it took a lot out of me just to stay with the pace. Six months earlier, I would have considered running Nicol so close in my first match against him as a great achievement. It was a measure of my growing confidence and ambition that I now regarded it as a disappointment. Once I had got over the shock of the first game, I thought I could win.

I returned home to take stock of the way the tournament had gone. It's sometimes difficult to judge your performance in a game immediately afterwards because you're still hyped up and emotional. A few days helps to add a little perspective. I watched my game against Nicol on video and was pleased with how well I had done. Even though I lost, it was probably the best squash I had played since I returned and I had to be pleased with that. After that first game there wasn't that much to choose between us. He finished stronger than I did, but I would have expected that. It was the first time I had played anyone of that standard for four years so it was bound to be difficult. I was delighted that I had adapted so quickly. If I had lost easily, I would have been disappointed and thinking that I still had a long way to go. But after 3–1 in a close match, I was confident I was getting very close.

Despite the jetlag and my efforts in New York, I felt quite strong when I got back home. That gave me a lot of confidence. Things were going well and I thought I could probably play in the British National Championships, which were only three days away. I tried a couple of practice matches just to make sure I really was okay and came through them with no problem. Ideally, I would have liked more time to rest before embarking on another tournament, but as I felt so good I decided to go for it. Perhaps it would be a good test for me to play two events back to back.

The tournament couldn't have started better for me. I got through the first three rounds without dropping a game. I hadn't really been tested, but I felt I was playing better than ever. I was seeing the ball early and hitting it cleanly. Then, in the semi-final, I came up against Paul Johnson again. The memory of our titanic battle in New York was still fresh in my mind. It turned out to be another marathon. This time I started the stronger and went two games ahead. It was probably the best squash I had played since making my comeback. I was starting to move a lot better and didn't feel so laboured. If your movement is good and you're getting into position early, that's half the battle. Unfortunately, it was too good to last. This time the tables were turned and it was my turn to tire after starting so well. He picked his game up and started to come back at me. He's a very hard player to put down, even when you're 2–0 up.

To a certain extent, my reputation might have been working against me in circumstances like that. Before I became ill, I was known to be a fierce competitor and very fit. If I managed to get 2–0 up it was enough to knock the fight out of most people. They knew I was very strong and there was very little chance of them coming back. After my illness, all that changed. People now felt that I became more vulnerable the longer the game went on because I was likely to tire at any minute. It gave them the encouragement to keep pressing when before they might have crumbled. I think this may have been in Paul's mind as he fought his way back.

He took the third game and came out even stronger in the fourth. He went quite a way ahead, and I could feel myself tiring. I realised he was in better shape than I was and I had little chance of catching him in that game. I needed a little time to summon up some more energy. I decided to ease off and take a bit of a rest. That meant effectively conceding that game and allowing him to level the match. It was a calculated gamble, because it might give him the momentum to storm his way through and win. Nevertheless, I needed that breather. It would give me the chance to refocus and hopefully come out stronger in the deciding game.

Paul took the fourth quite easily, as I expected. I knew he would be feeling confident that he could then go on and win. It was important to challenge that confidence as quickly as possible so I came out strong at the start of the deciding game. I stepped up the pace and started taking the ball earlier, as I had done in the first two games. I think it took him by surprise a little and I quickly built a good lead. That gave me the confidence and momentum to keep going. I think I probably played a little too fast for him and was able to take the match.

It was fantastic to win against such a good player, but I took equal satisfaction from the manner of the victory. I had played some of my best squash to go 2–0 up. It was disappointing that I let it slip but that was balanced by the fact that I was able to retrieve the situation. Sometimes, a match can take you by surprise and start to slip away just when you thought you had it under control. It had happened to me against David Evans in the British Open. I wasn't able to retrieve the situation in the game against Evans, but I had this time, and that was very satisfying. Those are decisive moments, when you find things out about yourself that you can't discover in training or with any amount of practice. It was like another little landmark on my road to recovery.

After the match against Johnson, I had a massage to relax my muscles. I had a good meal and then just tried to rest as much as possible. I wanted to make sure I would recover for the next day. My opponent in the final was David Evans. I had only been on the circuit six months and already I was playing him for the third time in a major competition. I was looking forward to it. I was still annoyed with myself for losing before, and wanted to put things right. I felt very confident. I knew it would be a hard match but I also knew that I was now playing much better than I had in the British Open. Then, I had won the first game comfortably but immediately lost my way and allowed him back into it. I was determined not to do that this time. I wanted to start strongly, as I had in that opening game, and then maintain the same pace throughout the match. I was confident he wouldn't be able to cope with that kind of pressure.

I knew more about Evans's game now. He's one of the tallest players on the circuit, so I would have to be very accurate when going cross-court or he would be able to play a good drop volley. He also liked to use a lot of deception. Sometimes he wouldn't hit the ball straight away; he would stop his swing and force you to pause on the T. Then he would hit the ball quickly leaving you a little flat-footed and struggling to reach the ball. I wanted to keep the pace up and rush him so he wouldn't have time to do that. Hopefully, I would be physically strong enough to do it. That would partly depend on how well I recovered after my long game against Johnson. I couldn't be certain until the following day.

I knew as soon as I woke up the next morning that everything was going to be fine. I felt physically strong despite the tough five-setter against Johnson. The two hard games in New York had probably helped me by conditioning my body to cope with that kind of effort. It gave me that extra bit of confidence and I was sure I would do well. I felt very focused. David Campion agreed to help me during the game, offering encouragement and pointing out where I might improve or exploit my opponent's weaknesses. It was a big day for David. His wife Cassie was through to the women's final, so he would also be helping her. David and Cassie were good friends of mine and I had been best man at their wedding a few years earlier. I asked David how he thought the two finals would go, and he said the bride and the best man would win.

The women's final was on immediately before the men's so unfortunately I couldn't watch Cassie play. In my first few tournaments, I had watched as many of the other games as possible but now, having reached my third final, I wanted to keep out of the way and focus on the task in hand. You need a break or it can get a bit draining. Cassie came through a topsy-turvy game to win 3–2, so the first part of David's prediction had come true. Now I had to do my bit.

I felt very good when I came out to warm up. Some people said afterwards that they could almost feel the concentration coming out of my head. The match went very much to plan. I came out hard and fast and I think David had trouble dealing with the pace. I took it 15–9. The second was even more conclusive, 15–6. I went 6–2 up in the third and then perhaps started to lose a little concentration, or maybe David just upped his game a little. Whatever the reason, he suddenly surged forward and took an 11–9 lead. That was a good warning sign for me. I didn't want a repeat of my previous game against him, when I had let the match slip from a winning situation. I could have taken a breather as I had against Johnson and tried to save my energy for a fourth game, but I didn't feel any need to do that. Instead, I felt I had enough in reserve to go up a gear and increase the pressure on David. I pulled myself together and decided to step up the pace further still, taking the ball that bit earlier. It worked. I think David was surprised by my approach and he wasn't able to cope with it. I won six points on the trot, taking the third game 15–11.

I had won. I was the British National Champion. The crowd erupted. I think the fans were genuinely pleased for me after all I had been through and I sensed a huge amount of goodwill from them as I stood to acknowledge their applause. It was a wonderful and emotional moment for me. In a strange sort of way, it only then dawned on me where I was and what I was doing. The championships were held at the Manchester Velodrome. As I looked round after winning the final, I realised what a wonderful setting it was and what a fantastic tournament it had been. I realised I hadn't competed in the national championships for six years. That was one of the first thoughts that hit me as the crowd started clapping and cheering. I had first won in 1992 when I beat Brian Beeson. That had been a great breakthrough and gave me a lot of confidence. I made a lot of progress up the world rankings after that. Two years later I won again, beating Peter Nicol in the final. Sadly, because of my injuries and illness, I hadn't been able to take part again until now.

Looking around at the sea of faces in the audience and sensing the emotion of it all made me realise what I had been missing through all those years. It crystallised in my mind. I came off realising that it was 1994 when I last played this event and now it was the year 2000. Everything had an air of unreality. I could scarcely believe I was playing again after all those years in the wilderness. Winning that day meant so much to me, much more than Detroit or Pakistan, and probably more than any other tournament I had ever won before.

With other tournaments in the past I had felt excited, of course, but now there was something more; a sentimental edge, because of all I had been through. Maybe it was because I was performing in front of my home crowd in Britain and they were responding so warmly towards me. I got a bit emotional as I made my speech after receiving the trophy. I felt a strong need to thank all the people who had stood by me in those dark years. People like Jonah Barrington and Dave Pearson had never wavered in their support and always showed great faith in me. That kind of help had been priceless and I will always be grateful to them.

David Evans was very gracious in defeat and warm in his congratulations. There was support too from my old adversary Chris Robertson, the man who had ground me into the dust all those years ago when I was the new kid on the block. It was a harsh but necessary lesson, showing me the difference in class between a seasoned professional and a raw teenager. Chris was now David's coach and in his corner for the match. He was obviously disappointed that his man had lost but seemed genuinely pleased for me. He described my performance as awesome, and said it was just like watching me in the old days. It was a nice gesture and I was grateful for his support.

The mayhem continued for an hour or so after the game, with the presentations followed by TV and Press interviews. I had forgotten what it was like but felt I could probably get used to it again. David and Cassie were also there to congratulate me. It would have been nice to go out and celebrate, but we all had to be up for training with the England squad the next day so that was out of the question. They both came down to Nottingham a few days later and we all went out for a meal together. It was the first chance we had to really celebrate. It was a wonderful time all round, all the more so because it had been so long coming.

After a few days, when the emotion had subsided, I was able to look back on the tournament and assess its real significance. It was great to win, of course, but as much as anything I was pleased with the manner of the victory. It was much more satisfying than the way I had played in Detroit and even Pakistan. Then I had been winning, but hadn't been playing anywhere near the level I wanted to reach. I had to rely too much on adrenaline and determination. Now I felt I was playing much better. I still didn't feel I was the finished article and I knew I could get better, but it was still a huge improvement. It gave me great hope for the future.

My only regret about the tournament was that Peter Nicol and Martin

Heath had chosen not to play. That took a little bit of the shine off my victory but I understood their reasons. They were unhappy with the level of the prize money. Some people thought they were being too greedy, but I sympathised with their stance. Everything and everyone must have a value. If all the top players turn up for a tournament even though they think the prize money is too low, then what incentive do the organisers have to raise it? On that basis, the pot would never increase and the sport would never move forward.

It's impossible to say what would have happened had they played but the way I felt at that time, I would have fancied my chances against anyone. As it was, all I could do was compete with whoever was put before me. It would have been a harder tournament if Nicol and Heath had been involved, but even without them there was still a strong line-up. With world-class players like Paul Johnson and Simon Parke involved, it certainly couldn't be seen as devalued.

In a strange sort of way, Peter Nicol may have contributed to my victory even though he wasn't at the tournament. The fact that I was playing better was partly down to the game I had played against him in New York. It sharpened me up enormously and provided me with a very clear illustration of the standard I was hoping to achieve. To get the best out of yourself, you have to compete against the best. I was looking forward to honing my skills against him again over the remaining few tournaments of the season but, unfortunately, it wasn't to be.

Like all professional athletes, I take great care not to injure myself in training. It's important not to overstrain yourself and vital to stretch out properly afterwards. I observe all the usual precautions, but then I did something that makes a mockery of all the care you take. About a week after the British Championships, I slipped on the stairs at home and banged my chest on the banister. It was extremely sore so I rested to let it recover. Again, the irony wasn't lost on me. I was just getting into the swing of things after being out all that time and was laid low by such a silly injury.

It came at exactly the wrong time, because there were three good tournaments coming up; the Esso Flanders Open in Belgium, followed immediately by the Millennium Irish Open in Dublin. The Al Ahram PSA Masters tournament came a few weeks afterwards in Hurghada in Egypt.

I wanted to play them all. They all carried world ranking points and I also wanted to see how I would stand up to three big tournaments in quick succession. If it proved too much, I would have plenty of time to rest because the season was ending.

My chest remained very painful but I thought I could probably play if I took some painkillers. I came up against John White from Scotland in the first round in Belgium and found myself in a titanic battle. I came through in five sets but it was hard work. My chest was very painful, but there was nothing I could do except grin and bear it because I had to face Simon Parke the next day. My chest felt even worse the next morning. My efforts against John White had aggravated it and I wondered if I ought to see a doctor. There was no time.

I did my best against Simon but I was never really in it. My chest just seemed to get worse in spite of the painkillers. He beat me quite easily and I came off court wondering whether the problem in my chest was worse than I had thought. I came home for a few days, but it was the weekend so I couldn't get to see a doctor. I had to fly out to Dublin to prepare for the next tournament so I arranged to go to hospital there. They X-rayed it and told me I hadn't bruised the rib – I had fractured it. No wonder it had been so sore. There was nothing much they could do. I just had to let nature take its course and give it time to heal up. I withdrew from the tournament and flew home. It was very frustrating, but I had to accept I was just as prone to mundane injuries as every other player. The season just petered out after that but I wasn't too disappointed. A six-week lay-off didn't seem too serious compared with everything else I had been through.

There was still a lot to be pleased about when I arrived home to Nottingham and took stock. The year had flown by, a good indication of how much I was enjoying myself again. I had made tremendous strides in my first season back. I had come from nowhere to break into the top ten in the world. I was now ranked number nine. If I hadn't broken my rib and effectively missed those last three tournaments, I was sure I would have got much higher. I was the British Champion and had won two other world ranking tournaments.

On the broader perspective, I had jumped in at the deep end and made my comeback. I had competed with the best, fought some gruelling matches and come through unscathed. I was much stronger at the end of the season than I had been at the beginning. It was more than I could have realistically hoped for just nine months earlier and seemed light years away from those dark days when I thought I would never play again. I was looking forward to the new season and felt quietly confident that I could do even better. I would be stronger, more confident and would have much more time to prepare. Not only that, but I was battle hardened again. There were still times when I didn't feel that well. Even so, I had managed to get back to the top in one of the most gruelling sports in the world. I had to be doing something right. The main task from now on was to keep on doing it.

# POSTSCRIPT

Both the sports world and the medical profession have come a long way since I developed CFS in the mid-1990s. The illness is now better known and more readily accepted. Doctors are more likely to be sympathetic with patients and have a better idea of how to help them. Coaches and back-up medical teams are better at spotting the danger signs when players start doing too much. The Australian Institute of Sports says that 90 per cent of athletes suffer from overtraining at some time. Usually the problems are only minor, but there are some extreme cases, like mine, where people become seriously ill.

The Institute's doctors monitor athletes to spot the danger signs before things get too serious. They carry out blood tests and various other checks to ensure everything is as it should be. They also produce psychological profiles on athletes by getting them to fill out questionnaires about things like their lifestyles and sleeping habits. Sports bodies in other countries are starting to do the same.

Sadly, this kind of support was unheard of when I was younger. If it had been available at that time, then I might not have become so ill. At the first sign of trouble, I would have been able to consult specialists who would have known what to do. Instead, I had no option but to see ordinary GPs who had very little idea about what was wrong, because they had little experience of CFS.

It's good to see that things are changing, although it's come too late to help me. In my case the damage has been done, but there's no point in worrying about it now. The most important thing is to make the most of what is left of my career. Hopefully, I have a few more years left in me still and I'm determined to enjoy them. It means creating a whole new mindset. Before I became ill, I was desperate to get to the top. I was like an express train hurtling towards its destination. I thought nothing could divert me from my chosen track, but I had reckoned without CFS. That had no respect for my determination or my mental toughness.

Like many people who have been through a serious illness, I've come to see things differently. I have a new perspective about what really matters. I wasn't the first person to work too hard and I'm sure I won't be the last. It's part of human nature to strive to get better and climb higher up the ladder. Now, I'm not so driven to reach the top. I'm still ambitious, of course. Don't let anyone be in any doubt about that. I'm not here to mess about. I would still like to become world number one and win both the world and British Open titles. Who knows? Maybe one day I will. I wouldn't rule it out by any means, and I don't think many of my fellow professionals would either. I still fancy my chances against anyone, but I shall have to wait and see how things go over the next few years.

In the meantime, I measure my success in different ways. The most important thing is that I have my health back. I would never presume to say that I've beaten CFS. That would be tempting fate too much. I had a good period after coming back on to the circuit, but I can't be certain that my illness might not return and stop me playing again. Even now, I still have times when it affects me. It was like that during the summer of 2000. I was under the weather for a few months and my performances were hit. I was probably only about 80 per cent of what I could be and that's not good enough at the very top level. This was reflected in some poor results. I don't want to go too far down that road, however. It sounds like I'm making excuses, which is the last thing I want to do. It's important not to go to extremes either way. I don't want to get too excited when things are going well, or get too downhearted when they start going badly. Hopefully, I shall take things in my stride more from now on.

Apart from my health, the main thing is that I'm playing again. I may never be as strong as I was but I don't care. I'm back at work in a very tough business. Being able to do your job seems such a simple thing, and most people take it for granted. To me it's colossal. There's nothing like spending four years on the scrapheap to make you realise how wonderful it is to be able to go out in the world and earn your living. So much of your self-esteem is invested in being able to support yourself by doing your job. It hurts to have that taken away.

Being the best in the world would still be great, but now it's enough to be a good professional player. I would never have thought that years ago, but the traumas I've been through since have altered my viewpoint. There are still times when I'm not only fighting other players, I'm also fighting my illness. That's tough opposition and it's unrealistic to expect myself to be always getting to the finals of tournaments and winning titles. I would be putting too much pressure on myself if I tried to do that. It would be detrimental to my health. There are a lot of good players out there. The overall standard has never been higher. I have thought about this in great detail: I can either stop playing because I can't be as consistently good as I used to be, or I can carry on and accept my limitations. I think carrying on is the better option because, in spite of all the difficulties, I still love playing.

A lot has changed since I was the fresh-faced new kid on the block turning up at tournaments full of the wonder of it all. In those days, I was hungry and frightened of no one. I was looking for scalps everywhere, hoping to come up against the seasoned pros so I could chop them down. Well, now things have come full circle and I'm the seasoned pro. Everywhere I look, there's a new generation of fresh-faced youngsters who are every bit as hungry as I was. The difference is that they're looking at me as the seasoned pro who needs chopping down. And just as I tried to exploit the diminishing physical powers of people like Jahingir Khan, so they are now trying to exploit my frailties. It's the natural order of things, and I have no complaints. I relish the challenge and I still think I will win more than I'll lose.

Whatever the case, the main thing is to enjoy it, because it's a wonderful lifestyle. At the start of the 2000 season, I went to America for the US Open but also agreed to play some exhibition tournaments. I thought they would be fun and would get me around the country seeing the sights. After competing in the Hong Kong Open, I took a few days off relaxing in Thailand before returning home. I wouldn't have done that before. I would have concentrated on training and preparing for the next big event. That approach has its merits, of course, if you're focused purely on success but I now want to be more relaxed. I don't want the highs and lows of winning and losing to be so intense. It'll help me in the long run, although the downside is that perhaps it will make me less competitive.

But as being competitive got me into trouble before, maybe that's not such a bad thing.

No matter what happens now, I'm proud of what I've achieved. To return after all those years and get back into the world's top ten as well as becoming British national champion is quite an achievement. The main thing, though, is that I'm back where I belong, doing my job. Despite all the knocks, I'm still standing. That's what gives me the most satisfaction. Anything else is a bonus.

# DAILY SUMMER TRAINING AND COMPETITION PLANNER

On the following page is a typical summer training plan, used by Peter Marshall from 26 June to 23 July 2000.

| MON | TUES | WED | THURS | FRI | SAT | SUN |
|---|---|---|---|---|---|---|
| 26 JUNE<br>David Pearson Light Technical (a.m.)<br>Interval Ghost (p.m.) | 27<br>David Pearson Plyometric Circuit (a.m.)<br>Rest & Recovery (p.m.) | 28<br>Strength Session (a.m.)<br>Practice Match (p.m.) | 29<br>Paul Carter Light Technical Session & Movement Drills (a.m.)<br>Interval Ghost/ Pressure Feed (p.m.) | 30<br>Paul Carter Plyometric Circuit (a.m.)<br>Rest & Recovery (p.m.) | 1 JULY<br>Practice & Movement Drills Strength Session (a.m.)<br>Rest & Recovery (p.m.) | 2<br>Rest Day |
| 3<br>Practice & Movement Drills (a.m.)<br>Rest & Recovery (p.m.) | 4<br>Training Camp | 5<br>Training Camp | 6<br>Training Camp | 7<br>Rest Day | 8<br>Practice & Movement Drills Strength Session (a.m.)<br>Hill Session (p.m.) | 9<br>Practice & Plyometric Circuit (a.m.) |
| 10<br>Practice & Movement Drills (a.m.)<br>Endurance Recovery Session – Bike (p.m.) | 11<br>Strength Session & Plyometric Circuit (a.m.)<br>Hill Session/ Practice Match (p.m.) | 12<br>David Pearson Plyometric Circuit (a.m.)<br>Interval Ghost (p.m.) | 13<br>David Pearson Movement Drills (a.m.)<br>Rest & Recovery (p.m.) | 14<br>Rest Day | 15<br>Strength Session & Plyometics (a.m.)<br>Hill Session (p.m.) | 16<br>Practice & Plyometric Circuit (a.m.)<br>Rest & Recovery (p.m.) |
| 17<br>David Pearson Movement Drills (a.m.)<br>Interval Ghost (p.m.) | 18<br>David Pearson Plyometric Circuit (a.m.)<br>Practice Match (p.m.) | 19 | 20 | 21 | 22 | 23 |
| | | | Rest/Active Recovery | | | |